STATE OF MIND

MIND

HOW I RAN 36 ULTRAMARATHONS
BACK TO BACK WITH NO TRAINING

CHRIS THRALL

SERF
BOOKS

State of Mind

Published in Great Britain by Serf Books Ltd in 2020.

www.serfbooks.com

ISBN: 978-0-9935439-3-7

Design by www.serfbooks.com

Cover image by MRE Photography

Back cover image by Hazel Mansell-Greenwood

1 3 5 7 9 10 8 6 4 2

Contents

For Jenny

Chris Thrall

Chris Thrall was born in South-East London. He is a former Royal Marines Commando who served in the Northern Ireland Conflict and trained in airborne insertion and Arctic warfare and survival. In 2011 Chris wrote the bestselling memoir *Eating Smoke* detailing his descent into crystal meth psychosis while working for the Hong Kong triads. A qualified pilot and skydiver Chris has explored all seven continents and backpacked through every country in North, South and Central America. In 2018 he ran an ultramarathon a day the length of Britain to highlight the veteran suicide epidemic and in 2019 completed a quadruple ironman distance triathlon. Chris has firewalked over red-hot coals to raise money to work with street children in post-war Mozambique. He has driven development workers to India and back by coach and scuba-dived in the Antarctic Polar Circle. In 2001 the Finnish Nation awarded Chris their Second Level Commendation on the grounds of human generosity. With a degree in youth work Chris is a life coach, an addiction specialist and inspirational speaker. He lives in the UK and plans to continue adventuring, charity work and hosting his popular *Bought the T-Shirt* podcast.

Social Media

christhrall.com

patreon.com/christhrall

youtube.com/christhrall

brandnewtube.com/@christhrall

bitchute.com/christhrall

linkedin.com/in/christhrall

twitter.com/christhrall

parler.com/christhrall

facebook.com/christhrall

facebook.com/groups/christhrall

instagram.com/chris.thrall

pinterest.com/christhrall

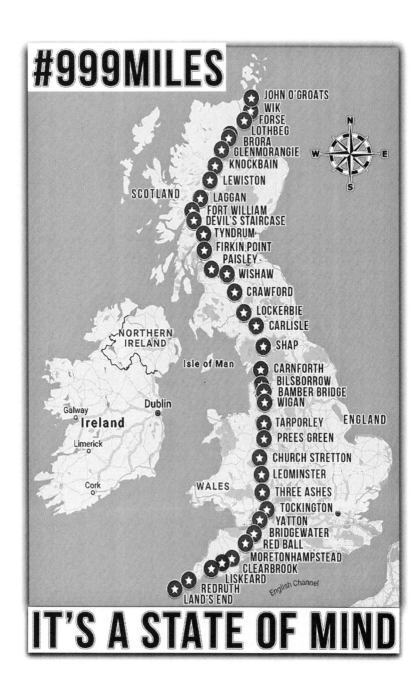

#999MILES

JOHN O'GROATS
WIK
FORSE
LOTHBEG
BRORA
GLENMORANGIE
KNOCKBAIN
LEWISTON
LAGGAN
FORT WILLIAM
DEVIL'S STAIRCASE
TYNDRUM
FIRKIN POINT
PAISLEY
WISHAW
CRAWFORD
LOCKERBIE
CARLISLE
SHAP
CARNFORTH
BILSBORROW
BAMBER BRIDGE
WIGAN
TARPORLEY
PREES GREEN
CHURCH STRETTON
LEOMINSTER
THREE ASHES
TOCKINGTON
YATTON
BRIDGEWATER
RED BALL
MORETONHAMPSTEAD
CLEARBROOK
LISKEARD
REDRUTH
LAND'S END

SCOTLAND

NORTHERN IRELAND

Isle of Man

Galway
Ireland
Dublin

Limerick

Cork

WALES

ENGLAND

English Channel

N
W — E
S

IT'S A STATE OF MIND

Author's Note

Some insignificant details have been altered for legal reasons. All references to medical information, medication, substance use, health, exercise, diet, training, planning and execution are purely to elucidate upon my own journey and mindset. They are in no way suggestions for others to follow.

An ultramarathon is any distance over 26.2 miles. By 36 ultramarathons back to back I refer to my average daily mileage. The longest distance I covered in any twenty-four-hour period was fifty-one miles across the final two days. I ran solo and without a support crew, carrying up to sixteen kilograms of food, water, equipment and camping gear. My mission was to raise awareness of the current veteran suicide epidemic and funds for the Baton charity.

Prologue

I've read a number of running books over the years and learned a lot about the various authors' motivation for lacing up their slog clogs – along with *every* mile marker passed on *every* event entered and *every* energy bar consumed. These inspirational individuals have achieved phenomenal levels of physical and mental fitness to become the stuff of legend and their memoirs are certainly engaging. Yet these somewhat two-dimensional accounts often overlook the psychosocial blocks the majority of us face when considering a challenge such as an ultramarathon.

For example, how do you entertain the idea of running a hundred miles when you're drowning in self-doubt, under pressure at work or battling the booze? What if you don't have time to train like Dean Karnazes or possess the plant-based culinary skills of Scott Jurek? Then there's peer pressure and society's glass prison. Why even contemplate an ultra-distance event when the sensationalist media would have you believe a half marathon is the domain of the athletic elite and your friends all shake their heads and go back to watching *Celebrity Toilet Swap*?

And where's the emphasis on implementing the all-important lifestyle tweaks that don't involve pounding the pavements and trails but are equally if not more important – alkaline living, mindfulness, gratitude, taking *action,* ultimate self-acceptance and a zero-negativity approach – easily adopted practices that can turn a mediocre runner into a super-achieving distance athlete who smashes all their goals?

As such I wrote this book for *you* – either to ratify the path you're on or provide encouragement and direction. There won't be any clichéd quotes, daunting training programs or silly words like hills, sprints and calories. I'll simply explain how by embracing adversity I smashed my ONE LIFE and how you can too with the right state of mind.

Respect,

Chris Thrall

Taking Action

A journey of a thousand miles ... is best undertaken
in running shoes.

Daisy Duke

The eerie black rock loomed out of the fog like something
from a Spielberg film. My lungs heaved, heart pounded,
sweat poured. A lifelong sense of failure fused with the
exhaustion and pain to suffocate me in self-doubt.

What the hell am I doing?

As I shuffled along the abandoned World War II airfield
in the dark, the idea of me joining an elite military unit
crushed down on the skinny shoulders of my 130-pound
frame. Upon spotting Helmstone Rock, a local landmark and
the halfway point on this excruciating one-mile 'jog', I sensed
my feeble spirit crash onto the potholed tarmac.

How can it still be that far? asked my exhausted inner child.
Why don't I just stop and end the suffering?

My pace slowed to *almost* a standstill ...

The demons closed in ...

How the insecure teenage me opted to act at this juncture
would change the course of my life. At forty-eight-years old I
would run 999 miles virtually nonstop, carrying a heavy
backpack and sleeping at the side of the road. Come forty-nine
I would complete a quadruple-ironman-distance triathlon.
Thirty years on I'd have explored eighty countries across seven
continents and achieved every single one of my goals. I'd carry
fire in my heart and peace in my mind, an enlightened

1

individual with the power to turn darkness into light.

New Year's Eve 1987 and I was unemployed and living in my car. Dan was my best mate. His father was a veteran of the Falkland's Conflict, a sergeant major in the Royal Marines Commandos, who on national television said of his South Atlantic experience, 'I took down boys. I brought back men.'

Upon leaving school Dan failed even more exams than I did. His options limited he decided to join the ranks of this elite amphibious assault force with its proud motto of *Per Mare per Terram,* 'By Sea by Land'. Dan was determined to earn the Royal Marines' coveted green beret, but before being offered a place on the gruelling eight-month basic training program, the longest and toughest in the world, he would first have to pass the three-day Potential Recruit Course at the Commando Training Centre in Devon.

The course hasn't changed much over the years. It is essentially a full-bore introduction to Royal Marines life combined with an assessment of whether or not you fit into it. A battle-hardened training team put you through some soft drills – such as making your bed in the morning and laughing at their crap jokes – and some hard ones. The latter involves a series of agonising physical tests designed to see whether your mind gives up or your heart does. They begin with an hour-long swim in the pool and as if this isn't challenging enough the Physical Training Instructor asks each potential recruit to fall backwards off the high diving board. With a mere ninety seconds to change into sports kit you then undergo a savage exercise session in the gymnasium, which sees lads spewing up, giving up or getting told their number *is* up.

As wannabe marines you spend the next couple of days wearing military fatigues and combat boots and having to complete a mile-and-a-half run in under ten minutes. After this comes the unimaginable exhaustion of the Tarzan High-Ropes Assault Course and infamous Endurance Run. Not including a four-mile jog to the start line, Endurance spreads across six miles of the Exmoor countryside, a treacherously hilly route interspersed with semi-submerged half-collapsed corrugated iron tunnels. Less than two feet across and up to fifty metres in length, these claustrophobic subterranean shafts are full of freezing cold muddy water, unforgiving stones, animal shit and even the odd snake. Needless to say, you have to drag yourself through without a second thought.

In training for real this involves carrying weapons and heavy fighting order and includes a four-mile run back to the camp's rifle range to place ten neatly grouped shots on a figure-eleven target – a Soviet-style soldier who fortunately at this stage in the proceedings doesn't attempt to fire back at you. This proves that you can run, keep your weapon in working order *and* shoot paper Communists.

Upon his return from CTCRM and having survived the ordeal with a pass, Dan scoffed with his usual dismissiveness, 'Of course, *you* could never do it!'

'Oh, you wanna *bet?*' replied this directionless young man, determined to prove him wrong.

I read Dan's glossy recruitment literature, paying particular attention to the fitness benchmarks required to pass the PRC. My dad had built me a climbing frame out of scaffolding poles for my fifth birthday. Complete with a military-like rope swing it was the height of our house, so the assault course and gym tests presented no problem for me. It was the running and swimming that could potentially be an issue.

As Dan and the rest of our buddies raised their pints to see the new year in, I slipped out of the pub, having made a deal with myself. *If* I could run to the Helmstone Rock and back *without* stopping, I would march into Plymouth's Royal Navy Recruitment Office after the bank holiday and sign on the dotted line.

Rumour had it Helmstone Rock was a meteorite that had crashed to Earth – although the more informed parishioners in this village on the edge of Dartmoor would tell you the thirty-foot-high black bulbous outcrop was actually igneous in form and the result of eons-old volcanic action. Regardless, I put my head down and continued grunting, panting and shuffling towards it.

In the cold, dark and mist the run and even *myself* faded into irrelevance. This wasn't about participating in a sports session and receiving a pat on the back for taking part. This was about combatting the all-encompassing urge to stop, as if the door of the recruiting office would slam in my face the moment I did. My sole focus was on not giving up – a stance in direct opposition to everything my jelly legs were telling me.

It was tempting to leave the road and take a short cut across the sheep-shorn grass, but I'd only be cheating myself. Instead I continued on the official route mapped out in my tortured head and finally rounded the enormous rock. Perhaps I should have experienced a runner's high at being on the home straight. In truth I was beyond sensing anything. I had nothing left in my mental and physical tanks bar the determination to prove my self-worth.

I gritted my teeth and pressed for home ...

An Unlikely Commando

When the going gets tough ... the tough simply figure if
someone else has done it then they can too.

Buzz Lightyear

As the train pulled up at the tiny platform, signalling the
start of thirty-two weeks of commando training, an
imposing red sign stood in stark contrast to the picturesque
boat-bobbing River Ex estuary scene stretching as far as the eye
could see.

LYMPSTONE COMMANDO.
Persons who alight here must only have business with camp.

Beyond the razor-wire fence spread the equally as
intimidating assault course, crawling with battle-clad recruits
like ants on the jungle floor. Past that stood several rows of
dazzling white three-storey accommodation buildings.

We wouldn't have the luxury of those six-man rooms yet
though. For me and the other fifty long-haired Lennys arising
from our seats it was the Induction Block for us, the
suspiciously empty bed spaces in the Full-Metal-Jacket-like
hall indicating five of our fledgling troop hadn't had the balls
to step off the train.

My three-day Potential Recruits Course had obviously been a
success – despite me developing an ear infection the week

before, perforating *both* eardrums, which meant I had to turn my pillow over each morning to hide the blood and yellow gunge from the corporal in charge. Although easily the hardest physical exertion I'd ever been put through I did okay in the swimming, quite well in the gym tests and found the assault course no problem. In fact, during my midpoint interview, the Women's Royal Naval Service officer said, 'Ahh ... so *you're* Potential Recruit Thrall.'

I wondered what gave.

'Did you *really* do nineteen pull-ups in the gym?' She grinned.

By now I'd gathered this was a good result. I'd manged twenty-nine in the recruiting office and still thought I'd failed. As it turned out the majority of blokes struggle to do more than ten.

The Endurance Course had been my downfall – or so I'd thought. I'd charged through the water obstacles and rocky tunnels and hadn't hesitated to be shoved into the eighteen-inch-wide seven-foot-long underwater culvert known as the Sheep Dip, trusting one of the lads to drag me out the other side. But on the four-mile run back to camp my skinny legs simply couldn't keep my waterlogged self up with the rest of the boys. I dropped increasingly further back until I was twenty metres behind and convinced the Royal Marines would say, 'Well done son, but try again next year.'

I couldn't let this happen. Not because I was determined to wear the green beret of an elite commando but due to the fact my long-since-divorced parents had told me I would never amount to anything and I had to prove them wrong.

'Alright, fella?'

As I struggled utterly despondent up the rocky track on Exmoor the voice came from my right. I looked up to see a muscular and moustached Royal Marines-type chap. Heartbroken I waited for him to tell me to stop there and that a truck would come and pick me up. I pictured the *gutting* train journey home and Dan's and my parents' gloating faces as I confessed to failure – at *life*.

'It's *frickin* hard, Corporal ...' I puffed, expecting him to scream at me, perhaps questioning my mother's wholesomeness or suggesting I had the ability to transit a golf ball through a length of garden-watering apparatus using only my lung power.

'Yes, mate, but you're doing *really* well.' He patted me on the back.

Huh!

'We're not looking for supermen,' he continued. 'We want guys like you – blokes who refuse to give up.'

Had I not been ballbagged *and* gobsmacked I would have said something. As it was I heeded his encouragement to catch the rest of the guys up and not long after our four-ton truck appeared around a bend.

'Right, *Five-Five-Eight* Troop, pick up your bags and follow me,' ordered our drill instructor, Corporal Smith, in a surprisingly pleasant tone. 'And don't try to march or you'll just look like idiots.'

As our oddball mob, all wearing various interpretations of 'smart', walked through camp in single file I felt like a French prisoner being shipped off to the penal colony. Little did any of us know this would be the only day in the next eight months that we would be allowed to 'bimble' anywhere. From here on in every recruit had to either jog or march around camp.

'Wai-eye, yorra canny blurk gerrin a logka necksta mee-lyke!' The recruit in the neighbouring bed space grinned through his acne.

What the hell did he say? I stared up at a chap who looked like Plug from the *Beano* – although that's doing Plug an injustice.

'I'm sorry?'

'Logka!'

As he rapped his knuckles on my 'locker' I gathered the guy was telling me I was fortunate to be in such close proximity to his handsome self.

'Oh … right. '

I was taken aback by this forthrightness. Up until now I'd been too unsure of my surroundings to utter a word. Even the electrical sockets could have given me an order and I would have jumped to attention, saluted and carried it out.

As my learning curve continued upwards like Evil Knievel's take-off ramp, I learned that this chap came from the species *Geordicus* and inhabited an area called Newcastle upon Tyne in the North of England – although why he spoke in a foreign language, I had no idea.

Belton was his name and finding out he'd spent several years in the Royal Marines Reserve, together with his obvious confidence, made me jump to the conclusion he was a *definite* candidate for the green beret. I shouldn't have done. For as amiable as Belton was as a person, he was a complete biff when it came to personal admin, not to mention physical exercise and fieldcraft – the sort of attributes that come in handy in a war.

On our Induction troop photo we sat in three tiers of chairs positioned on the parade square, all wearing our ill-shaped 'aircraft carrier' berets and looking like twelve-year-olds. Not long after our training team of four corporals, a sergeant and a lieutenant had pinned said picture to their office wall, Belton became one of the first recruits to have his face blacked out with a marker pen, having been sent packing for not making the grade.

Following on from having our heads shaved, being issued passports, signing on lots of dotted lines, swearing allegiance to the Queen and getting an introduction to the Royal Marines' unique inhouse lingo came the first gym session. Dressed in a green rugby shirt, white shorts and plimsolls we each stood on our allocated 'spot' (literally a white dot painted on the floor) in a huge gymnasium.

'Lie down!' screamed our physical training instructor, or 'PTI' a stocky handsome geezer in a red-piped white vest.

Half of 558 Troop dropped to the floor, while the rest remained standing and wondering what the hell he meant.

'Down!' he barked.

Before their arses hit the deck, *'Roll* over,' he shouted.

'Roll over!

'Roll over!

'Stand *up!*

'Sit *down!*

'Lie down!

'Roll over!

'Roll over!'

As I completed the seemingly simple task of rolling over I had never been so breathless – and this was only thirty seconds into the warm-up.

I was in for a double shockburger. Not only did the session expose a flagrant violation of the Human Rights Charter but as the PTI yelled, *'That* corner of the gym, *go!'* – pointing to a corner of the gym three miles away – my lungs ceased to function. A strange clogging sensation choked them, making me wonder if I might have undiagnosed asthma or something.

Of course, I didn't mention this to the training team and certainly not the sickbay. That would get me treatment on the spot – no pun intended – the 'pack your bags and go home, son' sort of treatment. I could never have that.

For although I was somewhat naïve, mildly introverted and far from the aforementioned superman, I had my sights firmly set on the day I would be presented a green beret, the mark of an elite commando, an achievement I could be proud of for the rest of my life.

Other than taking it one day at a time – what other way is there? – I had no game plan. I didn't even think about the gruelling challenges and tests that lay ahead. All I pictured was being awarded that prestigious green hat along with the accolade of 'Marine' Thrall. To be more truthful I pictured my parents and stepparents sitting in the audience in the camp's Globe Theatre in thirty-two weeks' time watching me receive it.

Having completed the arduous gym session without a whimper, figuring my chest problem was a result of the extreme anxiety our PTI intentionally whipped up, I found myself dressed in full-combat gear, minus SA80 rifle, being instructed how to put up a bivvy on Exmoor's gorse-swept Woodbury Common, an exercise not surprisingly named 'First Step'.

My bivvy partner for the two-day exercise was Hansen. I couldn't tell you much about Hansen because with fifty other blokes to get to know, all of whom heralded from places that definitely weren't Helmstone, I hadn't even had time to get to know myself. What I could tell you though was Hansen had a somewhat gentle comportment. His singing of lullabies while ironing as the rest of us drifted off to sleep in the dehumanising Induction Block in the early hours of the morning was appreciated by even the hardest men in the troop.

Hansen's softness was soon brought home to me. Because we didn't carry weapons on this non-tactical exercise – we weren't trusted to look after our own belly buttons at this stage in the program – the training team, who needed to familiarise us with a watch routine, came up with the bullcock scenario of 'fire danger'. Each recruit in their designated eight-man section would stand guard for one hour during the night to prevent the unlikely eventuality of Lucifer burning down the copse we were ensconced in.

After a day of learning how to feed, water and clean ourselves and our kit we crawled into our sleeping bags. One of the lads woke me for my pitch-black shift and ten minutes before the end of it I shook my bivvy partner expecting him to be lying there at the ready with one eye open, wearing his combat fatigues, fighting equipment and boots ...

Twenty minutes later Hansen emerged from under the canvas wearing only his Bart Simpson boxer shorts.

'Hansen, what *the* ...?'

It was obvious this kid operated on a different trip to the rest of us.

Needless to say our sloppy civilian-minded selves failed miserably at the morning inspection, with some of the guys' mess tins encrusted with enough of their ration pack to feed them through another day. Punishment was dished out left, right and Chelsea by the section corporals and one particularly bad offender, Sullivan, received the short sharp order to simply, *'Crawl!'*

Off Sully went on his hands and knees, across the clearing

and into the forest.

The kit muster went on for two tedious anxiety-inducing hours. By now the blistering sun was high in a cloudless blue sky. Just as we were attempting to cram our Aladdin's Cave of infantry gear back into our un-TARDIS-like Dad's-Army-style packs, *'Where's* Sullivan?' one corporal shouted.

Forty-eight recruits stared about them – but he was *gone!*

'We've got a *runner!'* screamed Corporal Pinkscarf. 'Let's go *get* him, men!'

On that cue our training team turned as one and charged into the undergrowth, giving the impression recruits often simply buggered off in the middle of an exercise.

The rest of us chased after them.

Opting for a sheep trail through the thick scrub, I jogged along for two miles, listening to shouts from the other guys. I was about to turn back when I spotted a pair of dusty combat boots dragging through the dirt and disappearing around the next corner.

'Sully, what you *doing,* man?'

Sullivan was a sickly grey colour, clearly exhausted and severely dehydrated, covered in dirt and twigs and bloodied by the spiky gorse and thorns.

'I'm crawling,' he replied from his trance. 'No one's told me to stop.'

During the week, we gathered on the enormous parade square, all wearing our half-lovat uniform and metal-studded brightly polished boots – or as bright as we could get them with our limited proficiency.

'Right, men, line out in order of your height, tallest on the left, and stand to attention,' Corporal Smith ordered, turning up an hour late having drunk four coffees to ease the pain of his hangover.

Shock number two – I *was* the shortest guy in the troop. Hell, I'd managed to go through eighteen years of life without realising five foot eight is pretty fucking small!

'Hansen, *prove!*' Corporal Smith barked.

Hansen looked up and down the line in the hope someone else shared his unassuming title. They didn't and so … *gingerly* he raised his hand.

'Report to the troop office *right away,*' the drill instructor continued.

As Hansen's toddler-like legs trotted his chubby body off, Corporal Smith turned to us. 'Men, take a *last* look at Hansen. Hansen is a *teddy bear,* and there is *no* room in the Royal Marines for *teddy bears.*'

Our second week in training saw us deploy on Exercise Twosome – 'Gruesome Twosome' as the more senior 'nods' referred to it. So knackered from physical exercise and limited sleep, recruits were nicknamed nods due to their propensity to fall asleep during lectures. Twosome plunged us – and our rifles – further into the business of staying alive in the wilderness and killing an *utterly* despicable enemy. We learned how to apply camouflage cream and live 'tactically' in the field, in addition to rationing our drinking water and keeping our bodies and kit in working order.

That night everything went *BANG!*

'Blank' rounds flew into our startled imagination from all directions, the gate-crashing training team screaming louder than your dad doing DIY. We were being 'bumped' by a highly inconsiderate yet pretend invasion force. As thunderflashes exploded and phosphorous-white flares soared into the night sky, my bivvy partner and I grabbed our equipment and legged it a mile to the emergency rendezvous point, 'ERV', a treeless mound known ominously as 'The Knoll'.

More lads arrived, frantic, out of breath and sweating off their camouflage paint, until the whole troop had regrouped. Some brought all their kit, some a part of it, some hardly anything at all. While we busied ourselves trying to make a shelter on the Knoll's inconsiderately steep slopes, the wind kicked up and bucketing rain began coming at us sideways. Needless to say it was a long and miserable night with little sleep.

Following a huge cooked breakfast in the comfort of their palatial and camp-bedded tent the training team arrived ... and they were *not* happy bunnies. In between the stomping and yelling these hairy-arsed potty-mouths emptied several kitbags brimming with combat gear – our *troop's* combat gear – onto the Knoll's windswept yellow grass. Fortunately no SA80 rifles dropped out – that didn't bear thinking about – but as sleeping bags, ponchos, clothing and other items of equipment tumbled onto the sopping wet ground, we knew a torturous 'beasting' was locked and loaded and labelled with our names.

Later in the day as the sun shone down, *'Right!'* screamed Corporal Flowers. *'Follow* me!'

He ran us at a sprint to the top of the Knoll.

'Fellas, it *pays* to be a winner!' he hollered and ordered everyone to descend.

'Winner' meant the first person back to the top got to sit down and relax while their compadres repeated the exercise ... *again ... again ...* and *again,* forty-seven times.

Knowing I wasn't the fittest horse in the race I adopted a middle-of-the-pack strategy, conserving my energy until I sensed I was the strongest bloke left. As I fought my way up the hill a tenth time I glanced left and right to check the extent of my fellow forerunners' grimaces. They clearly had nothing in reserve and so I put the power on and took my rightful place – on my backside – to watch thirty-seven more punishing attempts.

The next morning it was a sorry bunch of wannabe marines lined up in three ranks on Woodbury Common's infamous Heartbreak Lane. Unlike Exercise First Step, where we'd put on our issued Reeboks and ditched the heavy packs for a leisurely jog *halfway* back to camp, today would be different. However, I figured our first proper 'speed march', wearing boots and carrying eighteen kilograms of weaponry and fighting order, would prove a mere technicality and instead focused on the hot shower and delicious meal awaiting me back at base.

How *deluded* can you get?

By the time our long snaking concertina had covered half a mile I was way beyond any state of exhaustion imaginable, the fast pace even forcing one of the corporals to clamber red-faced – *more* red-faced – into the wrap wagon – and he wasn't carrying a rifle or equipment. The tarmacked road radiated the sun's merciless heat and this combined with the lane's thick and insulating hedgerows to create a four-mile-long sauna. For someone who'd barely sweated a drop during my limited pre-Lympstone training runs, I was soaked in seconds.

The chafing of the boots and webbing I could handle. It was the agony of maintaining a speed and stride way above my natural ability that was killing me. There was no way I'd ever give up though – yet this didn't stop me fantasising about collapsing onto the verge, thus providing a plausible excuse for bailing. A mile from camp, life had turned into one huge prayer, a plead to any god out there that Lympstone's perimeter fence would magically appear and end the insane agony.

'500 Metres to go. It's only PAIN!' announced a cheeky sign featuring a bulbous-nosed, shirtless and panting cartoon commando that some joker had nailed to a tree.

Pain didn't even begin to describe what I was going through. My poor little legs struggled to keep up with the troop and not throw my 'oppos' out of step – the last thing I needed was a chorus of wrath as everyone took their personal world of hurt out on me. The thoughts in my primate mind were: *Are we there yet?* and *Why the hell am I finding this so hard?* But my reptile brain clung to the simple logic that tens of thousands of young men had completed this march before me and therefore so could I.

When Corporal Flashard finally wheeled us off the road and into a field, I couldn't believe the torture was over. As the rest of the training team ran to save the life of a recruit who'd collapsed with heat exhaustion, 'Right,' said Flash. 'Stand up straight and breath in through your nose and out through your mouth.'

To this day I don't know if that technique works, for I was happy to lie on the grass breathing any which way I could – out of *any* orifice. I felt delighted to have completed the second week of training without drawing untoward attention to myself. I was painting the house ... one stroke at a time.

The speed marching continued to be the bane of my Commando Training Centre existence. With the exception of the Battle Swimming Test, I managed to pass every other physical, classroom and fieldcraft challenge with relative ease

– although 'ease' in the Royal Marines still requires one-hundred-and-ten percent effort, usually while hungry, wet, cold and yomping uphill. I was always second or third up the thirty-foot ropes and one of the two in the troop who could scale them wearing full battle order using only our arms - *twice*.

As the physical training progressed I learned to take things in my – albeit *limited* – stride and the asthma-like attack rarely resurfaced. I did so well in the gymnasium I received the accolade of PT Superior. Such was my agility when it came to doing 'regains' – which entails dragging yourself whilst wearing kit and a rifle along a horizontal hawser ten metres above a stagnant swimming pool, then purposely slipping off so that you're left dangling by your arms, before going through a six-phase drill to reclaim your position on the rope – I could skip all the stages and simply swing straight back into the 'commando crawl' in one fluid movement.

Not only was I the shortest guy in the troop but when the 'milling' came around I discovered I was also the lightest. Milling entails entering a boxing ring for three rounds and attempting to batter the bejesus out of the other fella. I scanned the fight schedule and breathed a semi-sigh of relief to find I'd been pitched against Recruit White, who I'd always assumed was the skinniest lad in 558. But when I checked the weights scribbled next to our names on the roster, I realised I was *two* pounds lighter! There was no dancing around the ring, no Muhammad Ali stuff, we just smashed the knobs off one another until the final bell. I was awarded the win but would be the first to say we both deserved it.

In Week 30 I finally nailed the swimming and so it was only my old nemesis the Endurance Course, along with three other commando tests, to complete. Of course, nothing is that straightforward in the toughest military basic training in the world. All of us were injured, many with fractured legs, and one lad, Fraser, undiagnosed pneumonia. I had Achilles tendonitis in my right ankle, so painful I chopped the stiffened leather from the heel of my boot to prevent it rupturing the ligament any further. We'd just stepped out of a ten-day final exercise, covering over a hundred miles carrying eighty-pound bergens to attack our final objective. This left the troop semi-starved and exhausted from minimal sleep under canvas in February's sub-zero conditions. To make matters worse the tests are crammed into five days, Endurance on a Friday, in between the Tarzan High-Ropes Assault Course and a nine-mile speed march. Come Monday we needed to complete a thirty-mile run across Dartmoor's snow-capped highlands in under eight hours.

At this stage everyone feared getting back-trooped for not making the grade. This would mean having to join the intake two weeks behind us. Worse still, if badly injured a recruit might end up in the remedial 'Hunter Troop', which often led to a medical discharge and the end of a young man's elite green dream.

Surprise-surprise Dan, who'd entered training a fortnight ahead of me, was ejected from 557 Troop and deposited into our Fighting 558. His bully of a sergeant had sought any excuse to bin him because Dan's father was now an officer. Nevertheless I was pleased I'd taken Dan up on that bet when I'd been living in my car eight months ago in Helmstone. It was yet another reminder never to measure yourself against another human being ... *or* their big mouth.

On the morning of our Endurance pass-out run I knew I had to pull something out of the bag. We'd had two practice attempts both of which I'd failed miserably, not even getting anywhere near the seventy-two-minute cut-off time. My problem was simple – I found running *incredibly* hard. Although agonising, I kept up when speed marching with the squad because to drop out would be letting them down. But on Endurance there *was* no squad. You started in a threesome because the second obstacle, the sheep dip, required teamwork. After that you were on your own.

When my alarm buzzed at 5am I threw on battle fatigues and fighting equipment and went to collect my rifle, joining the shivering group of lads queuing outside the armoury. *Jeeze* it was cold! Minus six, our billowing white plumes of breath making us look like a gathering of chain-smokers. Despite carrying twenty kilograms of equipment as we jogged up the narrow winding lane to Woodbury Common, we all knew this was nothing compared to the punishment ahead. Just the thought of charging into Peter's Pool's icy depths made me shiver.

'*Go!*' yelled the instructor.

Mick Cowan and Alan Dillon sprinted downhill towards the freezing river at a pace that either meant business or they were trying to kill me. It's a strange thing to plunge yourself into bitterly cold water without a second thought – you'd never entertain such insanity as a civilian – but in we went with our rifles above heads. Fortunately for our trio the teams in front had broken through the three-inch layer of ice, saving us valuable seconds as we waded across up to our necks.

Emerging from the shallows I watched the lads power off up the steep rocky track. My soaking wet bitterly cold clothes and kit now weighed almost double as I slogged after them. By the time I reached the sheep dip Mick and Al were in our pre-arranged positions. Without pause I laid my SA80 on the concrete bridge and dived into the narrow underwater tube like an obedient torpedo, relieved to feel Mick's hand grabbing my webbing as he hauled me out the other side. Having carried out the three-man evolution we were off, me in the soul-destroying position of being last ... *again.*

I crawled through the rest of the waterlogged torture chambers as fast as I could, a check of the watch confirming it was my slowest time yet. Upon hitting the road for the four-mile slog to the rifle range ... my spirit departed and my legs turned to lead.

The reason the Royal Marines training is the hardest in the world is because it truly is hard ... *extremely* hard. I simply had nothing left to give. I broke into a walk, resigning myself to the fact a career in a military elite obviously wasn't for me.

Then came my saving grace ... in the unexpected form of Recruit Manson. Manson was a back-trooper who'd proved to be an even worse runner than me.

'*Come on,* Thrall, *we* can do this,' he yelled.

The irony of the troop's worst physical asset having to encourage me hit a nerve. I couldn't let Manson reach camp first, not when he'd started three minutes after me. I checked my Casio. I had thirty-two minutes to complete the test, which meant running at an eight-minute mile pace. It seemed an impossibility. I'd only ever run an eight-minute mile in PT kit and certainly couldn't envisage doing it weighing as heavy as a tank.

I stared down the tarmac. Was *this* it? Would I let eight months of gruelling but successful training go out of the window?

I suddenly experienced an overwhelming sense of self and all I was capable of. I began putting one foot in front of the other, building to a jog ... and *then* I let rip.

Until the excruciating pain of fatigue slipped me into unconsciousness I would damn well *run* – and that's what I did.

Upon reaching the camp's main gate I'd caught up with Mick, chasing his heels all the way to the target range. *'Thrall!'* inquired our gobsmacked officer, stopwatch in hand. 'Did you start off with *Cowan?'*

'Yes, sir!' I puffed.

Mick had obviously made the cut-off time … and so had I.

A Funny Thing Happened Down in Chinatown

*Ask not what your country can do for, but where can
you buy a Nutribullet.*

Mahatma Gandhi

Serving in the Royal Marines had been a blast. After receiving my green beret I was posted to 42 Commando in Plymouth. Not surprisingly my first run there had been a disaster. You'd think after thirty-two weeks of commando training I'd be as tough as old nails. In truth I was totally drained. We set off in sports kit on a 'gentle' five-miler and I immediately began to struggle with the six-minute-mile pace. Approaching a Tesco supermarket my brilliantly sharp mind came up with the inarguable excuse I needed to evacuate a chocolate hostage. I peeled off from the pack ... and walked my useless legs and miserable self back to camp.

I served with merit in the Northern Ireland Conflict, a particularly bloody five months during which we were sniped at and bombed on a weekly sometimes daily basis, one of our brothers shot dead in the first fortnight there. Following this I arrived in the north of Norway to commence three months of Arctic warfare and survival training. I'll never forget putting on a ninety-pound bergen and skis for the first time, promptly slipping on my arse and figuring this had to be a practical joke.

Having sailed around the world for fourteen months as part of a twelve-man high-security detachment on board the aircraft carrier HMS *Invincible,* I arrived at Plymouth's Stonehouse Barracks to commence three years of soul-destroying guard duties. I'd had a phenomenal time in the Royal Marines but felt it was time to move on.

Along came a business opportunity marketing consumer-electronic products. Hooked immediately I began building an international distribution network in my free time. The day I left the military my company had turned over in excess of a hundred thousand dollars, mostly in Asia and so that was where I was headed.

Hong Kong! Bright Lights! Big City!

The Pearl in the Orient was one *hell* of a place to be ... the only issue being the £3,900 a month I'd once earned, a veritable fortune in 1995, had fizzled to nothing. The company supplying mine with products had collapsed, leaving me in a bustling commercial hub filled with seemingly infinite opportunity ... without *any* opportunity. Plus I was £8,000 in debt.

Hong Kong is the business capital of the world. Steeped in ancient and exotic culture and a unique mix of Anglo-Sino history it's hands down the most incredible place on Earth – bar perhaps Plymouth or Torpoint. Picture a vast emerald-green harbour crisscrossed by every type of enterprising craft imaginable, from traditional sampans and antique red-triangular-sailed junks to multimillion-dollar yachts, state-of-the-art hydrofoils, hulking-great cruise and container ships, all weaving an intricate web of commerce with their frothy white wakes. Imagine a jagged waterfront skyline of mirrored-glass skyscrapers rising with impunity into the cloudless blue azure above Central District like a lineout of powerful financial Goliaths.

Embrace the heat of tropical Asia as it drenches you in sweat the moment you leave the faux-comfort of your air-conditioned building. Witness the surreal humidity in monsoon season as well as the ferocity of the cyclonic monsters that whip through the colony, sweeping rubbish bins, street signs, palm trees – and anything else not tied down – horizontally along flooded streets. Stand amazed as the Met Office beeps a hurricane warning signal to the pagers of eight-million people simultaneously, all of whom immediately cease swinging their umbrellas around on packed streets or leave the office to rush home and barricade themselves in a tiny cramped apartment. In grids of thousands these rabbit-hutch-like frontages bely the most expensive property rates in the world.

Immerse yourself in the chaotic raucous throng spilling onto crowded pavements from gold-and-red-fronted establishments embossed with eye-catching Chinese-charactered signs, shops selling anything from Cartier to rhino horn. Experience vibrant market places where frogs and snakes writhe in tubs alongside racks of poultry and slabs piled high with butchered beef and pork, not to mention baskets laden with pak choi, lychees, pineapple and every other exotic food fayre imaginable.

Sit yourself down with a litre-bottle of beer at an open-air restaurant to sample steaming noodle dishes, deliciously cooked chicken, crab, lobster and other enticing platters that make you realise the takeaway menus back home are a salt-and-sugar-laden joke.

Then there's the mysterious superstition and rigid etiquette, once hidden behind a great wall, a vast desert and an enormous mountain range, but now either clashing, complementing or reconciling itself with the West. Craggy faced five-foot-nothing grandmothers dressed in traditional black cotton garb and wide-brimmed straw hats rush along pushing rickety wooden carts piled high with rubbish bags from restaurants. Old men looking wise and reserved in tailored cheongsams, skullcaps atop long plaited hair, who following the appropriate introduction will predict your fortune by reading the lines on your palm.

And did I mention the infamous Wan Chai nightclub district, home to the Legend of Suzy Wong, where pounding disco music booms from neon-flashing doorways? Filipino bar girls work the wallets of jawing American sailors. Wide-eyed tourists wander the pavements wondering what they are letting themselves in for. A raft of expats and entrepreneurs head with distinct purpose to their favourite drinking hole for a Jack Daniels-and-Coke or a bottled Latino beer.

I loved Hong Kong, immersing myself the culture, wolfing down the cuisine, befriending locals and expats alike and busying myself learning the language. Having bunked in with 'Vance' Lee Hok Keung, my amazing Chinese business partner, in a rat-infested outhouse tagged onto the back of his apartment, I took a job selling computer components in an old-school Chinese trading company, Gung Wan Hong, only I got sacked for daring to speak Cantonese. With so much money at stake in the computer chip business our wily old boss didn't want a foreigner understanding his international dealings in case I syphoned off some trades.

I got a job selling advertising space in a business publication that ... *didn't* actually exist. Fed up with the endless bullshit of money-making and not wanting to waste my young life away in a suit, I returned to what I knew best, *security,* and took a job as a nightclub doorman. Only, the demons of a traumatic childhood had yet to have their say and before I knew it I was hooked on crystal meth. The first time I inhaled the vapour from this harmless-looking heated-up translucent rock I felt utterly amazing, filled with abundant energy and an ultra-positive attitude towards life.

Two months later it was a different story ...

My behaviour became so erratic my dear brother Vance kicked me out of the flat. I slept rough until a sign saying 'Pawn Shop' enticed me into selling my Rolex and I used the thousand pounds to rent a shitty top-floor flat in a decaying tenement in a rundown part of Wan Chai. I took a job working for the 14K, the notoriously vicious triad gang running the area, as a doorman in the sleazy Club Nemo. My fellow bouncers were Dai Su, a six-foot-six assassin, and Chu Chi, a hard-as-fuck streetfighter.

Off my bonce on meth I was in the market one day, seeking to buy bedding for Apple, a Filipino working girl who'd moved in with me. I picked up a blanket in a shop ... *and my world changed forever.* For the rough grey cover in my hand was *obviously* one of those infected with tuberculosis the US Army had given to the indigenous American Indians in an attempt to wipe out the population as the White Man moved further West. I was *stunned* that this shit was taking place before my very eyes in *Wan Chai* of all places, in *modern-day* Hong Kong?

What the fuck was going on? Was this some sort of conspiracy? Perhaps a *global* conspiracy?

I looked at the shop assistant – and *she* averted her eyes.

I glanced at the guy standing at the street corner – and *he* did likewise.

Fuck! How could I have been so *stupid,* so *blind,* my *entire* life!

Whatever this weird underground plot was it encompassed my mind for the next five months. I began a meticulous process of examining any literature at hand – instructions on food packets, slogans on billboards, articles in magazines – in attempt to crack the cipher and gain entry into this bizarre double world. As for physical fitness I danced all night in the Big Apple and chain-smoked knocked-off Marlboro supplied to me by my hard-nut triad brothers. Crystal meth made me feel *brilliant,* the person Mother Nature *intended* me to be and not the ostracized kid I'd always felt.

Then one night it came to a head in the club. The more my fascination with this ancient criminal fraternity increased, so did their suspicion of me. That I spoke the language made them even more wary. One of the triad bosses' girlfriends had 'accidently on purpose' bumped into me as I stood on the door tapping my feet to Two Unlimited's 'Tribal Dance'. *'Pok gai, gweilo!'* she spat – *gweilo* meaning 'foreign devil' and *'pok gai'* the highest form of Cantonese insult.

Rather than take the bait I laughed and told the moll I didn't understand Chinese, which infuriated her even more ... *or* so she made out.

Before I knew it the 14K's bouncers from nearby establishments began spilling into Club Nemo, all with menacing black eyes and comments of 'We're gonna kill you, *gweilo!'*

Life ceased to be fun. These guys seriously had a bone to pick with me – and I envisioned my own agonising death as they drew their ferocious chopping blades.

Everything went white ... *silent* ... *sterile* ... and I knew I was about to die.

And then I *laughed!*

Stupid fucking triad *wankers!* Who did they think they

were intimidating? I was a Royal Marines *Commando*. I'd stared down the barrel of IRA guns *and* laughed my ass off as I did. I wasn't afraid to die – *only* of being a coward. *Fuck 'em!*

I readied myself for the fight, secretly daring the first chancer to step forward so I could punch his deluded head in …

I had no idea what that shit in the club had all been about – only that I'd survived. I'd lost everything, my military career, my money and possessions and, for all I knew, my house back home. I hadn't paid the mortgage in months. On top of this all my so-called friends had disappeared. There was only one thing for it – I had to crawl along a wire cable, one spanning Jaffe Road to the building opposite mine. I had to see the fat lady sing – the big girl's silhouette appeared every night in the swirled glass pane opposite. It looked like a microphone in her hand – although to a non-mental person it was most likely a hairbrush. If I could shin along the wire in the darkness, doing the commando crawl, and reach that building everything would suddenly make sense and I would prove I wasn't the worthless loser everyone thought I was.

I laid my body onto the wire and *crikey* it was high, the cars in the street below looking like toys. But I *had* to do this thing. Not only was it the moment my Royal Marines training had conditioned me for, but also when I reached the other side the complex façade shielding this weird global conspiracy would fade away, revealing the true meaning of life and my purpose in it.

I began inching my way across the abyss, determined to prove to the haters I possessed ultimate belief in myself and they could all go and fuck themselves.

But then I stopped …

Swaying there in the darkness, seventy metres above a potentially horrendous demise, I thought about my dear little brother, Ben, back home. He wasn't aware of this Hong Kong nonsense encompassing my tortured world – bosses who'd fired me, triad assassins and expats stabbing me in the back. He only knew his heroic big brother, a role model who'd surmounted our challenging upbringing to become a rough tough *Royal Marine,* was in Asia making a go of his life. I loved that little bro, my only friend when our parents separated for the umpteenth time and we'd ended up hundreds of miles away at yet *another* strange school. If I fell to my death Ben would live the rest of his life under the belief I'd fallen foul of drugs in the Far East and thrown my sorry self off a skyscraper. I *couldn't* let that happen.

I stopped my commando crawl, swaying there, alone and staring down at the miniature street scene below. *What* was I trying to prove and *who* was I trying to prove it to? I didn't care for those sneaky two-faced expats or tattooed blade-wielding thugs. And if there was a worldwide conspiracy then whoopy-*frickin*-do! I only cared about my dear kid brother, my best friend, and I didn't have to prove myself to anyone ... except him.

I thought about the handsome fourteen-stone bodybuilder who now weighed less than ten. I thought about driving my BMW to give business presentations in top hotels and the smart new house I'd bought at twenty-three.

Where it had all *gone?*

I wasn't a *bad* person? Sure, I had my faults like anyone else, but in truth I loved and respected everyone – even those who'd turned against me. Whomever this drug-zapped shell of a human being was I didn't deserve to end up in this unbecoming state.

And with that a wave of emotion swept over me. Tears began running down my face and dropping into the abyss like paratroopers from a Herc. I struggled off the wire and returned to my pigsty of an apartment, sinking down amongst the clutter of taken-to-pieces appliances, ant-infested food wrappers and stale drinks cans to cry like a child.

When the Virgin Atlantic flight touched down at Heathrow my own father – now confused and traumatised himself – didn't recognise me. Dad had covered the airfare. He had also paid some of my mortgage payments and managed to rent the house out, yet I was still thousands of pounds in arears. As I sank down on the sofa in my two-bedroomed new-build my family were simply happy I was home.

I was far from it …

There was a gaping hole in my heart at having to leave my beloved Hong Kong, my *true* home. I missed the incredible culture, the people, the food and the language. I longed to work on the door again and practise kung-fu in the park at 7am. Had the medical world been on the ball they would have diagnosed chronic depression and complex life-long trauma. As it was they told my father I was suffering from severe psychotic illness and recovery was unlikely. They suggested admitting me to a secure psychiatric facility to live out my days.

I couldn't care less about professionals who hid behind clipboards and attempted to fob me off with happy medicine – all of which I chucked in the bin. Despite several more run-ins with the police, adding to my not-so-impressive Hong Kong tally, there was *nothing* wrong with me – nothing a healthy dose of base amphetamine couldn't fix.

Before long my immaculate house was as smashed up and

bloodstained as that crummy apartment in Wan Chai. On the plus side that weird 'inner voice' had long-since gone. But as I began shoving filthy needles loaded with ridiculously strong speed into the fragile veins of my ever-skinnier arms nothing really improved. I was signed off work indefinitely – not that I had the self-belief or qualifications to even get a job. Utterly depressed after four-day sleepless binges I'd lie on the sofa wrapped in a filthy sleeping bag and watching crappy daytime TV. My meals consisted of pasta shells mixed with porridge oats, milk, margarine and sugar, because my addicted mind only ever kept a quid or two back to purchase a fortnight's food.

Despite the enormous undiagnosed black cloud looming overhead this was my mad mental life and I lived it without complaint. The speed would sort things out. *Surely* it would. After all it was the wonder drug that helped me find my true self in Asia ...

At times I became so desperate I tried reaching out to past acquaintances, but with a look of utter shock in their eyes they'd say, *'Christ,* Chris, *what* happened to you?' I had no money for proper heating and my emaciated body suffered from hypothermia so badly I kept a hairdryer in the front room to stop me lapsing into unconsciousness and a slow death. I developed itches all over my skin and became utterly convinced the house was infested with lice. I ripped up the carpets and burned them along with my clothes and bedding in the back garden, then submerged myself in a freezing cold bath mixed with bleach – I couldn't afford to put the immersion on even in winter.

And then one day everything changed ...

I'd woken up clad in only my boxer shorts whilst wondering

who I was and where I was. Shivering on the bare floor I could hear the kids playing in the street. I was the only adult in Carroll Road who wouldn't tell them to get lost for having a kickaround outside my front door. I was starving and hadn't eaten for days. I wanted to slip on my filthy clothes and nip to the corner shop to buy a pasty with my few remaining coins. But the second I stepped out the door the kids would come running and ask me to shoot penalties or similar. They loved me those kids. I always treated them as equals and would never subject them to the draconian violence my cohort suffered whilst growing up.

Realising my life had descended into such dishevelment and chaos that I was too ashamed to leave the house hit home hard, the sunlight beaming through the blinds reminding me there was a world of possibility out there I no longer felt a part of.

What the hell have I done?

I cried for hours, for all the hurt I didn't deserve as a kid, and when I finally stopped whimpering I embraced the rays of light reaching down into my damaged world ... and I *smiled*.

It was time to rebuild my life ... *one day* at a time.

I wouldn't be going to any support groups or praying to a god – I wouldn't even change my lifestyle. I'd simply moderate certain areas and get some balance back into my routine.

I grabbed my world globe and circled all the countries I wanted to explore, making a mental list of every activity I wished to experience along the way. I would earn my pilot and skydiving licences, take an advanced scuba-diving course and explore the Antarctic Polar Circle. I'd dive off the cliff in Acapulco like my hero Elvis did when I was a kid and catch piranhas in the Amazon. Hell, I might even write a *book!*

Before that though I would complete a world record

firewalk to raise money to go and work with street orphans whose lives had been torn apart by years of bloody conflict ...

I was going to *AFRICA!*

A Very *London* Marathon

If you love yourself, run a mile. If you respect yourself,
run a marathon.

B.A. Baracus

Catering to the children's unique needs made surviving
malaria, dysentery and Mozambique's forty-degree heat
more than worthwhile. When evening fell I would leave my
co-workers drinking tea in the security of our small cliff-
front compound and visit the nearby village. In amongst the
mud huts I'd down coconut shells of hooch, smoke the local
ganja and dance to drumbeats around the campfire with the
tribe. I soon sacked off the notion that sub-Saharan Africans
needs overly privileged White folks to develop them – the
NGOs appeared to profit from their sustained poverty – and
instead went fishing and swimming with the kids in the
turquoise waters of the Indian Ocean and hitchhiking
around the war-torn country.

While on my six-month service in the scorching sun two
life-changing events took place. First I struck up a
relationship with Hanna, a beautiful Swedish team mate
who I'd met on the training program back in Norway, and
then the humanitarian organisation asked me and another
English guy, Lee, to drive fifteen volunteer journalists to
India and back in an old school bus, our mission being to
write magazine articles about communities living in poverty.

Norway, Sweden, Denmark, Germany, Austria, Italy,

Greece, Turkey, Iran, Pakistan, India *and* back again, it truly was the trip of a lifetime, and leaving the merciless desert heat, incredible scenery and Bedouin and bandits to drive a twelve-ton coach into the heart of Delhi's crazy traffic was something I will never forget.

Following this I fileted salmon for ten months in a Norwegian factory on a small island called Frøya near the Arctic Circle. I used the money to backpack around the world, through every country in North, Central and South America as well as most of South-East Asia, Europe, Australia and New Zealand. Having enrolled my uneducated self on a university course I began studying for a degree in Youth Work, using the generous end-of-term holidays to continue to tick items off my bucket list.

After our summer sabbatical in 2004 the lecturer asked each pupil to tell the class what they'd been up to for the past eight weeks. 'Trips to the beach,' said some. 'Barbeques and pub,' announced others.

... I kept quiet about attending flight school in Florida to undergo pilot training and upon receiving my licence flying an aeroplane twenty miles up the coast to Sebastian to embark on two weeks of mad mental skydiving. I said nothing about hanging out with homeless Vietnam veterans on Miami South Beach before jetting to Mexico to grab a flight to Cuba, where I learned all about Castro's revolution and spent a day with one of Che Guevara's former rebel commanders. Nor did I mention backpacking through El Salvador, Columbia, Venezuela, Guyana, Surinam *and* French Guiana, camping out in the Amazon rainforest and catching piranhas to eat.

The following summer I explored Israel and Palestine and visited New Zealand, Singapore, Malaysia, the Philippines,

South *and* North Korea and Japan. But along with travelling there was something on my mind ...

The London Marathon.

During my three years in the wilderness of addiction the only running I did was to meet drug dealers. In Mozambique I'd revived my long-overlooked and somewhat spiritual pastime, often jogging along the paradise-like beach and then plunging myself in the ocean to prevent heatstroke. Come winter 2004 I hadn't run since Africa four years previous, having been so caught up with life my fitness got pushed aside.

Anyone who watched *Blue Peter* as a kid will recall Peter Duncan's drama-laden London Marathon attempt. The program's young audience was invited to submit a design for his running outfit – and *boy* did he look a dick! Back then the marathon represented the peak of physical fitness and mental endurance. As such, stowed away in my never-say-never mind was the dream I would someday pit *myself* against the 26.2-mile challenge.

2005, I decided, was going to be the year.

I'm not sure why – I was terribly unfit and partied for days on end at every opportunity. Plus if I announced my plan to family and friends they'd reply, *'Why* do you want to do that?' or *'You'll* never do it.'

Everything I'd ever achieved in this life was off my own back and usually contrary to others' negative input. The London Marathon would be no different. I applied for a place through the annual ballot but when November 2004 rolled around, six months before the big off, my application hadn't been successful. I had the option of running for a charity though and chose an organisation providing rehabilitation to drug-addicted prisoners.

Next I flew to America to secure a pair of leading-edge running shoes along with some state-of-the-art vitamins and advice from three former New York Marathon champions ...

No, I didn't. Without changing into anything particularly 'sporty' I laced up my shagged-out Asics and half-ran half-walked ... around the block.

Why?

Any exercise no matter how short infuses you with a sense of achievement. You've taken *action!* Having eased yourself over the first – often intimidating – hurdle the subsequent endorphin rush leaves you feeling incredible. But if you set your unfit-self up for some overly ambitious five-miler you can end up talking yourself out of it or resorting to the walk of despair.

Pretty much everything I've accomplished in adult life – whether it be shaking off the depression of inactivity or completing a life-enhancing course – has begun with a quarter of a mile jog. It's the best medicine Mother Nature has to offer and it's free. My quarter-mile blast signalled the start of my marathon adventure. Before long I was upping the distance to a mile, then two and more.

Training is addictive and it's tempting to run every day. Your body needs time to rest though and so I would do two short distances during the week and a longer one at weekends. Initially it took me thirty-six minutes to cover three miles – far from the pace I'd managed in the marines. I'd write down my finishing times – as there's nothing like slicing a few seconds off a previous best to spur you on to continue.

One day I drove to Dartmoor for a bit of cross-country.

There was a light rain, the air crisp, the ground hard underfoot. I jogged along a sheep track, skipping around gorse bushes, hopping muddy puddles and ducking under low-hanging branches to avoid having the headphones ripped from my ears.

Then it suddenly hit home – the *unique* aspect of the marathon!

You see, it was *me* doing this. Along with thirty-thousand others *I* was the one who had the self-belief to make *my* dream come true. And yet with this investment comes a great deal of uncertainty. Six months' training simply isn't long enough to 'breeze' twenty-six miles.

I was vaguely aware four hours is considered a respectable marathon time, because it means you've run nonstop and pushed through the infamous pain 'wall'. At this stage though my sole aim was to complete the race. The literature suggested newbies shouldn't attempt the full distance during training due to the long-term damage this has on the body and the subsequent recovery time. Apparently you should aim to peak at the twenty-mile mark about three weeks before the event and taper from there. The additional six miles will be gifted to you on the day by the Marathon Fairy – a combination of adrenaline, commitment, a roaring crowd and London's relatively flat course. But it's one thing being told you'll be fine crossing into this unchartered territory, quite another living with the uncertainty for months.

I began to feel a soreness in my right foot. Upon inspection I found the peroneal tendon was clicking over the ankle bone each time I took a stride, the result of a severe sprain in the military. I bought a neoprene strap which worked more as a placebo than support. Then something happened that changed my life forever, the most important discovery I've ever made, the simple secret to life-long happiness, balance and success.

I'd been suffering from what I thought was giardia, having picked up the minute but havoc-wreaking stomach parasite while trekking in the Andes. I took several courses of antibiotics but the upset continued for months. I provided stool samples to my GP and underwent an endoscopy, all of which showed negative for the bug. Then I happened upon a newspaper advert offering anyone suffering long-term ill health the chance to have their blood inspected for abnormalities. I met with the specialist, Nathan, who turned out to be a microbiologist and a pioneering authority on something called 'alkaline living'.

I'd only begun to pay attention to my diet in 1995 after attending a three-day seminar by the world-famous life coach Tony Robbins. Having taught his audience to walk across red-hot coals Tony went on to expose the myths and food-industry propaganda supporting capitalism's toxic cuisine. Yet despite making changes – consuming way more vegetables and a lot less meat, dairy, caffeine and sugar – I continued to come down with colds several times a year as well as an annual bout of the flu.

As I stared at a huge TV screen displaying my live blood sample, 'Acid, Chris,' said Nathan, referring to the white blobs floating amongst my ill-shaped red blood cells. 'What was the last thing you ate?'

'Bowl of All-Bran.'

'That'll do it.' He nodded knowingly. 'Refined carbohydrate.'

Nathan explained how each item of food or drink we

digest has an effect on our blood's PH level, which should ideally average out to 7.25 across our lifespan. He gave me a book, *The PH Miracle,* which further elucidated upon this fragile balance that *all* of the world's 'diets' fail miserably to comprehend. Our hunter-gatherer biology evolved over hundreds of thousands of years to live in equilibrium with the ecosystem. Sure, the 'paleo' way of eating recognises the *type* of food human beings require to thrive but it doesn't acknowledge the all-important *ratio* they should be consumed in – as would have been dictated in the natural environment by the four seasons of our climate.

Humans thrive on chlorophyll – sunlight turned to energy. By placing a focus on acid-producing meat and likewise carbohydrates at the expense of alkalising ingredients such as vegetables most people's bodies are in a constant state of acidosis, the root cause of most ill-health.

To be clear here, we're not talking about whether you buy organically grown produce from Marks and Sparks. We're referring to the 'spoonful of peas' or 'lettuce leaf and a slice of tomato' on the side of the plate scenario that's become the unhealthy norm in cultures the planet over. Although far from essential to human health, animal protein and carbs are okay in moderation but your meal should always be two-thirds greens or a similar alkalising produce or else the fragile tissues, the *ecosystem,* within you will remain toxic and eventually lead to disease.

I bought some PH testing strips to check my saliva. The result was shocking. Instead of a healthy green the indicators turned red, a sign my body was way too acidic, hence why, like most of the country, I was ill so often. I modified my food intake and began drinking a litre of vegetable-and-lemon-juice smoothie a day, adding heaped spoons of 'super greens', a vegetable-rich powder. After a day or two my body began to detoxify and boy was I in for an eye-opener! With years of toxins suddenly dumped into my bloodstream I felt *weird,* as if on a hallucinogenic drug. I went for my weekend run and managed a hundred metres before walking demoralised back to the car. My legs had turned to lead.

But as the side effects of the detox wore off a metamorphosis took place. Not only had the hip pain I'd been suffering vanished but also the soreness in my ankle. I hit the road for a hilly three-miler, expecting the usual breathlessness and heavy legs to start off with ... but these previous handicaps had *vanished.* Instead I sprinted the whole way and knocked *seven* minutes off my personal best. In that moment I suddenly understood what it meant to be a *proper* runner, in mind and body, as nature intended – *and* my stomach problem had cleared up.

Nathan was right. I could see now that for my whole life I'd blindly bought into the multi-billion-dollar disinformation campaigns funded by the food and medical industries. The notion you can defy the laws of nature and alter your body's all-important PH balance now seemed as ridiculous as watering your pot plants with Coca-Cola and thinking they will flourish. I incorporated this one-third-meat-and-potatoes two-thirds vegetables philosophy into my diet and haven't had so much as a sniffle in seventeen years.

The London Marathon is pitched as 'The Greatest Race on Earth' – but it's so much more than that. In 490BC a Greek messenger named Pheidippides ran from the Battle of Marathon 26.2 miles back to Athens with news of their

Persian enemy's defeat. Legend has it that upon bursting into the government chamber he announced, 'We have won!' and promptly collapsed and died as a result of his superhuman effort. However, contemporary science has shown how over-exposure to endurance running can lead to heart problems, so it was more likely a lifetime of long-distance telegraphy led to our hero's demise.

The first marathon race took place in 1896 at the inauguration of the modern Olympic Games in Athens. It was won by Spyridon Louis, a Greek water-carrier, in two hours and fifty-eight minutes – the *slacker*.

Then a magnanimous Olympic Commission let *women* enter the event – a swift *ninety-eight* years later! It was America's Joan Benoit in the 1984 Los Angeles Olympics who crossed the line for the double-first in two hours and twenty-four minutes. The oldest annual marathon, the Boston, began on 19 April 1897 and the New York City race in 1908, marking the start of the running craze known as 'marathon mania'. But in 1981 former Olympic track champion Chris Brasher, Roger Bannister's sub-four-minute-mile pacemaker, and Olympian John Disley, a three-thousand-metre steeplechaser, founded the London Marathon, its pioneering runners crossing the start line on 29 March.

The London Marathon changed the face of the event the world over, turning it from a competitive meeting of highly focused athletes into a city-wide carnival. Here indomitable Britain's historic and multi-cultural heartland the age-old adage of 'It's not the winning, it's the taking part' truly came into its own. Whether you are an ultra-tuned athlete from the sands of the Sahara, a ninety-year-old pensioner up for an eight-hour 'sprint', a marathon virgin or a charity-minded philanthropist dressed in your wife's underwear, the London will welcome you whole heartedly. Everyone who witnesses the spectacle goes home a better person for it. There is no greater experience – with the possible exception of the *EastEnders* omnibus or finding the missing piece for 'Kitten in a Handbag'.

Two weeks before the big event my training ended with an unintentional twenty-two-mile bimble out to Dartmoor – *sans* water bottle or bankcard. Upon reaching the picturesque Burrator Reservoir, *Bloody hell!* I thought. I'd run a half-marathon without breaking a sweat and remained unfazed by the nine miles home. The human body is an amazing machine.

Halfway into my return journey dehydration forced me to beg a glass of water from a café along the route. However, as this lean mean running machine set off towards the city … the 'lean, mean and running' functions no longer worked. My legs had seized, but determined not to break my 'no walking' rule I pushed through the wall. I was in *agony,* absolute *agony,* but a hot bath and a cup of tea more than made up for it.

Not training for a fortnight before the event was a great decision, for despite drinking way too much beer the night before I felt raring to go on the day. Following a complimentary cuppa at the starting point on Blackheath I hugged my buddy, Stuey, and went to join the mass of excited amateur runners (the professionals and wheelchair warriors get under way from a different location) forming a half-mile-long throng. I located my entry point as dictated by the guesstimated four-and-a-half-hour finishing time I'd written on the application form and slid in amongst the charity

Rhinos and sports-shoed superheroes.

As I stood there taking in happy faces, terrified faces and possibly suicidal ones, the starter's pistol fired and we were *off!*

No ... we weren't.

Our merry band of adrenaline junkies, many removing bin-bag bodywarmers, didn't budge an inch. It was five minutes before we even began shuffling towards the start and another fifteen to reach it.

But then we *were* off – and it was brilliant!

Thirty-thousand distance-divas waved at the BBC camera on the gantry overhead and began chasing down the race favourites – Kenya's Martin Lel, Morocco's Jaouad Gharib and South Africa's Nelson Mandela.

Approaching a small park, I saw long lines of runners queuing for portaloos. I had no intention of screwing up my marathon time and so joined the boys taking a hasty leak on the grass.

Two hundred metres on a sweaty and deathly-white middle-aged man loitered on a patch of wasteland. Attempting to look nonchalant, he was obviously calling his wife to come and pick him up. Be wary of drunken New Year's resolutions is all I'm saying!

The way ahead quickly became blocked by the deluded Johnnies who'd overestimated their abilities when filling in the application form. I kicked myself for being too conservative and wished I'd slipped in the starting lineout nearer the front. To skirt the logjam, I began running *behind* the spectators lining the curb.

It's funny to think a marathon is simply running along the road, because the London is *so* much more. Spectators from all walks of life come out in their thousands to cheer you – a complete stranger – on. Some of the well-wishers' attentions get distracted by the numerous pubs dotted along the route, but most people stand five-deep on the pavement, clapping and shouting *your* name – if you've written it on your shirt that is. I could hear '*Go on,* Chris!' 'Well *done,* Chris!' 'In the *bag* now, Chris!' from these good kind folks as they looked me sincerely in the eye.

And it's not only the adults who've got your back – the kids are amazing too. They stand in the gutter, holding their hand out for a high-five – not always easy to reciprocate in your exhausted state. Many of the children hold up bowls, like little Buddhists pleading for alms. It's the other way around though because the receptacles are filled with jelly babies. But twenty metres further on you see these sickly treats stamped into the tarmac – no one has the appetite for sweets a mere five miles into the race.

I continued forth, relaxed in my stride and weaving round the ten-minute milers, all the time scanning the cheering masses for Stuey. But as we'd never agreed a meeting place a reunion was *never* gonna happen. This was a shame because I looked forward to having a familiar face acknowledge my efforts.

Stu was likely in one of the pubs, all of which blared out booming rock music. Apparently Paula Radcliffe's husband had called all the landlords during the week to request they play Tina Turner's 'Simply the Best' as she ran past. This was a great strategy, for as I'd found during my training, music provides a much-welcomed adrenaline boost – although if Paula was being spurred on by such an inspiring tune ... surely her *competition* was too?

Ordinarily I'd listen to music while running in an event – despite a lot of organisers prohibiting the use of headphones on the grounds of safety. On the London however, an MP3 player is unnecessary due to the cheering crowd and the aforementioned rock music. In addition a variety of musical acts set themselves up in convenient spots along the route. Yet it soon becomes apparent that many of these cats are there to hear their own meowing. Who wants to hear 'Sweet Caroline' performed by a pub singer when your in a world of pain? It has the opposite effect of the Rocky soundtrack, making you want to run over and strangle the chancer with his own guitar strap.

The London is an amazing day and you're made to feel like a celebrity, a champion and a *marathoner* all at the same time. To win the event must be incredible, akin to performing to an adoring crowd at Knebworth. Another unique feature of the race is London's iconic landmarks, places you may have only seen on the box. The first was the *Cutty Sark,* an immaculately restored clipper, a veteran of the China tea trade and one of the fastest sailing ships ever built. After you've carefully navigated the majestic craft's cobbled dockside so as not to turn an ankle it's four miles to Tower Bridge and the glorious experience of crossing this impressive span under the glare of TV cameras.

I checked my watch to find I'd run a half-marathon in well under two hours, leaving me on track for a sub-four-hour time. I still felt as fresh as a daisy, in complete contrast to breathing out of my arse only five short months ago. I felt good, *super* good! Nineteen miles in, following a cold shower from the overhead sprinklers set up on Canary Wharf, I was still full of steam.

... Nineteen and a half miles in and I found myself in *Hell,* not helped by a demoralising stretch where the course turned back on itself. In an instant my energy vanished, legs turning to concrete as I hit the dreaded wall, the only positive being I was now heading along the Thames Embankment towards Buckingham Palace, not far from the finish. Approaching the twenty-three-mile marker, the long-established Lucozade refreshment point, I knew Johnny Wilkinson the England rugby legend would be handing out drinks ... only as I arrived he was deep in conversation and had his back to the course.

'Johnny!'

'Well done, fella!' He grinned and gave me a bear hug.

It was a massive boost from a kind-hearted man, one I'll never forget. I surged onwards along the river, even breaking into a sprint ... for one hundred metres. Then I tripped on thin air and only just managed to rescue my tottering self.

The crowd went *wild!*

That last three miles was harder than the Royal Marines' Endurance Course. What with me hitting the wall good and proper my dreams of a sub-four time fizzled into nothingness.

Who was I kidding?

I slowed to a walk, resigning myself to completing the race outside of the all-import four-hour cut-off, the line between serious marathoners and jokers dressed as Batman.

Attempting to take it easy proved to be a saving grace, for my legs had completely seized and I was unable to walk. In so much pain I manged three paces before resigning myself to a less-agonising trot.

I checked my watch – ten minutes left to complete the last mile. *You can do this, Chrissy!*

My pace quickened.

I forced my aching body along Birdcage Walk's strangely pink tarmac, utterly spent as I passed Buckingham Palace and the Victoria Memorial. I had no idea where the finish actually was, but hitting the Mall I saw the sight I'd always dreamt of – the Flora banner signalling the end.

My suffering instantly disappeared. I sprinted the last three hundred metres to thunderous applause. I had no idea if I'd achieved a sub-four, because the digital clock over the line read 04:22:02, the *official* race time. I just made sure to click the stop button on my watch.

As I hit the rubber-matted walkway there was no throwing of arms in the air. I simply slowed up and glanced at my G-Shock.

Three hours and *fifty-six* minutes.

It was one of the proudest moments of my life.

I'd bloody *done* it!

Smiling at the Morning Sun

Shit happens...

Shuey McFee

The next ten years can only be described as 'all good character-building stuff', to use a marine's parlance – 'something of a nightmare' in everyday terms. It started in 2006 with a phone call from Sweden. Hanna my girlfriend called to update me on her mother's lung cancer, saying she only had a week or so to live. My stepdad Dave had been battling leukaemia for the third time in his life. A stem-cell transplant gone wrong had resulted in the disease eating him down to the bone. Dave didn't complain – not once. He ended up in a wheelchair, face bloated out of all proportion from the steroids, his limbs as thin as broom handles.

Hanna was nine years younger than me and our relationship had experienced endless upheavals as a result of this incongruence and our countries' often opposing social norms. After Hanna had relayed her mother's deteriorating condition, I gave her an update on Dave's situation. 'But he's *only* your *step*father!' she snapped and hung up.

I knew at that moment the girl I'd loved dearly for seven years and had travelled around the world with, indeed *thought* the world of, was gone from my life. I put the phone down and rather than endure the usual end-of-relationship depression, made a decision to never think about her ever again.

I wasn't being cold-hearted – in fact the opposite. Our

mental health is incredibly fragile and it needs to be managed with a firm set of hands. I'd already spent almost two years of my life debilitated by the black cloud and was never going there again. My relationship with Hanna was never going to work. We'd had an amazing time of personal growth together, but everything has to end at some point and now we were a step closer to finding the right person for ourselves.

Besides, I think it's important to learn how to be content on your own and not let a partner, a job role or an exclusive club define who you are, thus stroking your ego and facilitating a phoney sense of happiness. Like a Samurai warrior I compartmentalised the event and then smiled at the morning sun and cracked on with my life.

Hanna's mum died three days later, Dave just before Christmas, a week after that. After I'd closed this gentle giant of a man's eyes, giving him the peace he deserved, particularly after such a long and unfair battle, the morphine pump kept clicking, injecting the now-redundant drug into Dave's lifeless body via a cannula in his thigh. My brother turned the little machine off and I removed the needle and emptied the remaining medication down the sink. Being a former commando and a combat-trained medic, I didn't think twice about this last act of respect for the man I always called 'Dad'.

This is where things got complicated in the way only family and grief can. My mother and siblings got the wrong end of the stick and accused me of stealing the morphine to go and get high on. The next thing I knew not only was I dealing with the ending of *two* close relationships, *plus* a – soon-to-be – chronic relapse into addiction, but I had my mum on the phone telling me I was the 'most disgusting person' she'd ever met and banning me from attending the funeral. Fortunately my good mate Dave saw the truth of my predicament and drove me to the service, where I was able to say a few words in Dave's honour.

I'd been doing well in my studies of Youth and Community Work at Marjons University in Plymouth. Now though, as I attended lectures while juggling a major drug problem – not to mention a full-time job – everything began to slide the way of the pear.

Come evening, so ragingly high on amphetamine, I'd drink twelve cans of strong lager and chain-smoke spliffs just to get into a position to even think about sleep. Then I'd lie on the bed wide awake until four in the morning, nodding off for two hours before the speed in my system woke me up. Huddling under the duvet, cold, shattered, anxious and alone, I'd have to inject the drug into my arm just so I could face getting out of bed.

Upon arrival at university I'd neck a beer, stub out a spliff and head for the gents' for another hit of the strong stuff before my first lecture. A few concerned eyes would raise from folks who'd been there themselves and who could tell from my bloodshot eyes and dilated pupils I was holding onto life by an edge. I never complained though. This was *my* wonderful life and no one ever said it should be easy. I would make the right decision when necessary. I always did.

The problem was I found myself with a submission deadline and an essay not *quite* finished. Rather than hand in sub-standard work I went to see the university's counselling service to bluff a chit for extenuating circumstances – thus receiving an extra two weeks to complete the assignment. The woman I saw sat *smoking a cigarette,* while attempting to pry into my personal life. All I wanted was for her to sign my excuse notice so I could bug the hell out, but instead she said,

'So, are you going to come for another session?'

Shit! I didn't care to be here for *this* session let alone return for another. I only needed a signature. Rather than appear a lead-swinger, 'Yeah, book me in,' I replied.

When I arrived the following week the wicked witch was ill and so I saw an elderly Geordie chap not surprisingly called ... *George*. His understanding manner was the polar opposite of Esmerelda and I had no problem telling him a little about my life, such as serving in the Royal Marines, surviving the Hong Kong triads and experiencing addiction.

'Well ...' He sighed.

I waited for a pearl of wisdom.

'I've *got* to be completely honest ...'

'That's good.' I smiled.

'I've ... I've never *met* anyone like you. You've lived *ten times* more than me, and I *don't* know if I can help ...'

I braced for the clincher.

'But ... I will *damn well* listen!'

This kind old Geordie being so frank was one of the most therapeutic things I'd ever experienced. I saw him another four times. He never really had any answers but always kept his promise to listen – and sometimes that's all you need.

On our final session George leant forward and tapped me on the knee. 'And you should give this *running* malarkey a miss. At thirty-three you've got to take care of your body.'

I grinned.

There wasn't a hope in hell's chance I'd ever quit such a life-giving sport ... but I didn't tell George this.

In the summer my best mate Lee asked if I wanted to go on a road trip to Portugal to a psytrance festival called 'Boom'. Lee was from Manchester. He'd been my co-driver on the bus trip to India and his love for life matched mine. We bombed down to Portugal in a brand-new Lexus owned by Nigel, a wheelchair-bound friend of Lee's. En route, in the playboy resort of Biarritz, Lee and I went for a dip in the sea.

'I thought you couldn't swim, Lee?'

'Been teaching myself.' He grinned.

We had a splash in the invitingly warm water, Lee doing something that resembled a doggy paddle – although that's doing the canine community an injustice.

The following afternoon the three of us arrived at the festival, only it didn't start until the next morning and so like the hundreds of other party goers we pitched camp on the shore of a beautiful lake. After a couple of beers we made our way to a gazebo on the beach where a couple of mad DJs were belting out thumping tunes. A random French guy approached wearing pinstriped trousers that gave him the look of a court jester. He and Lee fell into conversation and a few minutes later my buddy turned to me and whispered, 'Ketamine?'

'Did you do some?'

I already knew the answer to both our questions.

Lee winked.

'Why not,' I replied, figuring horse tranquilizer was exactly what we needed on top of forty-eight hours with no sleep.

I snorted a line off the back of the guy's hand.

The party had *definitely* started! I found myself going from knackered traveller to disco king in seconds. As I connected shapes in the warm moonlit night, Lee nudged my arm. 'Liquid acid?'

I looked over to see Monsieur Pinstripes waggling a small brown eye-dropper-type bottle.

'Did *you* do some?'

Lee grinned.

I wasn't a fan of LSD, a drug that can induce long-term psychological damage in certain individuals on the first time of taking it. Looking around the shoreline of this idyllic lake though, I could see loads of funsters with these small brown vials and, not wishing to miss out on what a psytrance festival is all about, I decided to indulge.

'Just a *drop!*' I told the jester.

I'm not sure if it was the language barrier or perhaps naivety but the guy *drenched* my hand.

'*Whoa ...!*' I shook a load of the potent liquid off and took a tiny dab with my tongue, conscious the hallucinogenic chemical was soaking through my skin.

Then I blacked out ...

I don't know how long I was unconscious, but I awoke to find myself lying on a patch of stones by the water's edge. I heard a groan and saw Lee collapsed three metres away. 'Lee, you alright, man?'

'*No ...*' he moaned.

Fuck!

Not only were we incapacitated but the world had shifted sideways. My body no longer worked and I found myself on an alien planet where the laws of physics didn't apply. Of further concern, the party continued on around us with everyone seemingly oblivious to the seriousness of our predicament.

I struggled to my feet and conducted a customary check of my pockets – phone, wallet, tobacco, lighter – making sure there was still a Rolex on my wrist. 'Lee, get up, dude. We're going back to the tent.'

Another hour was lost, for the next thing I knew we were back at the party gazebo. The tsunami of incapacitation had evaporated, leaving me feeling out of this world as if I'd landed on Planet Hedonism. Everything seemed wonderfully surreal – a billion light years beyond brilliant – and mere words could never encapsulate the experience. Not only were colours, shapes and scenes not doing what they were supposed to but my fellow ravers were all so unbelievably friendly, supplying me with endless hugs, water and cigarettes. The men all looked so handsome and the women damn gorgeous. One stunning Spanish girl took a shine to me and we danced, smiled and kissed. I was literally in heaven in a parallel universe.

Lee seemed fine at first, wandering around sporting a huge grin. After a time though, I noticed he was mumbling to himself and his lips were cracked because he probably hadn't drunk any water. 'Mate, you okay?' I went to put my arm around him.

Bam!

'*Whoa ...!*' I recoiled.

His *head butt* landed just short of my nose.

'Lee, calm the *fuck* down!'

Assuming Lee was still coming around from our ordeal I got him to sit down, but the second I turned my back he was up and *running* towards some poor Portuguese chap, who he then *rugby tackled* to the ground!

I dived in and split them up, but the guy was obviously far from happy. Fortunately he and his mates understood Lee was having a bad trip and didn't beat the shit out of him – no matter how many times he lunged at them like a mad dog. They could see I was having a nightmare trying to take care of my mate. I had no other option. Nigel had gone back to the tents, but even if I managed to get Lee back there he'd never sleep, not in this wired state. Plus the second I took my eye off him he'd get into god knows what trouble.

The whole scenario was a huge great awful contradiction. On one hand I was having the best night of my life – Lee's erratic behaviour aside. As the sun appeared over the horizon stacks of funsters threw off their clothes and when for a dip in the shimmering lake. Jeeze there were some beautiful Latin girls going to this festival, one that threw open its entrance gates in four hours' time.

On the other Lee had overdone it *as* usual – not that I held a grudge. I loved the guy. Lee was my dear mate – one I had driven halfway around the world with. He just enjoyed getting *extremely* high. On the usual party prescriptions this had never been a problem – although I always worried that he would do himself some harm. Now however, it was different.

'Lee *behave* mate. Stand there and *dance!*'

I hoped the effect of the acid would soon wear off. But even in my ultra-tripping state I was beginning to wonder if there was more to this than Lee being off his head. Maybe he was having some sort of a psychotic episode?

When I next turned my back he was off, charging through the tents, which spread a mile along the shore. I wasn't sure what to do. I'd lost count of the number of times he'd attacked me. Maybe I should wrestle him to the ground and put him in an arm lock ... but *then* what? How long would I have to sit on him before he regained his lucidity – that could be twelve hours or more?

People were packing their gear, ready to join the long queue of vehicles heading to Boom. I began asking some of them for help, but no one would take me seriously, so I ran back to our car.

Nigel sat behind the wheel rolling a joint.

'Mate, we've got a problem.' I panted. 'Lee's lost the fucking plot.'

'Ah fuck him.' Nigel concentrated on his bifta. 'He always gets fucked and ruins everything. Let's just go to the festival.'

I was confused.

I wasn't sure if Nigel understood how serious the situation was –

Wailing sirens broke out ...

Blue lights erupted ...

A police car hammered down the rocky track to the lake, skidding onto the shore and driving flat out across the beach. *Another* followed ... then *another* ... and *another* ... *two* ambulances in the rear. The scene was surreal, the emergency vehicles shattering the peace of this lakeside idyll and replacing it with terror.

'Fuck ...' I shook my head. 'He's dead or he's killed someone.'

'*Shut* up ...' Nigel sneered. 'Let's go to the festival.'

Just as I began to tear into the selfish idiot a slim olive-skinned girl approached the car. "Ave you guys got a friend 'ere?' she asked in a French accent.

'Is he dead?' I replied.

''As 'e got a tattoo on 'is leg?' she continued.

'Is he dead?' I pressed.

'Er ... you should *just* get down to the lake.' She shrugged her helplessness.

Nigel attempted to start the Lexus, only him listening to the stereo all night had flattened the battery.

'Wait here. I'll go,' I said.

Tripping my face off I commenced the longest walk of my life, knowing Lee's dead body waited to greet me – you don't need six emergency vehicles for a case of sunstroke. As I made my way along the water's edge the remaining campers stood in silence, most projecting a look of condolence. When I reached the first ambulance the driver leant against its door, the other emergency vehicles clustered nearby.

'Is my friend dead?'

The paramedic looked at me and nodded, his eyes flicking to a blue plastic sheet ten metres from the gently lapping waves.

I walked over and lifted it up.

Lee's lifeless eyes stared up at me.

'You *fucking* idiot ...' I muttered.

I bent down and kissed his forehead.

When I retired to a rocky outcrop to roll a cigarette a group of young locals walked over. 'It's your friend?' one man asked.

'Yeah, his name's Lee.' I shrugged.

They all took it in turns to give me a hug.

'We see Lee struggling in the water,' said the chap. 'We rush in to save him. But ...'

He went on to explain how they'd tried to resuscitate my friend to no avail, shaking his hands to emphasise how awful it had been.

We swapped email addresses.

Five minutes later a woman from the TV news approached, a cameraman in tow. 'Can you give us an interview?' She thrust a microphone into my face.

'No ...' I waved my hand and walked away.

The police seemed remarkably nonplussed – as if this sort of thing happened every day. By now the scorching-hot sun was high in the sky and my skin had been burning for over an hour. The news woman kindly went to her car and grabbed some sun cream. The cops asked me to attend an interview in the police station in the nearest town, Castelo Branco.

Making my way back to the car I briefly wondered if it was time to hang up my party clogs – but would Lee say if he could hear me talking such nonsense?

'Man up, *wanker!*' is the answer to that one.

This was simply a terrible accident. Lee had drowned. I wasn't going into victim or blame mode. If you use recreational drugs there's a chance of dying. Lee and I had known that and willingly accepted the odds.

Nigel had got the car jump-started and met me en route. Peering through the windscreen, he mouthed, 'Whaaa ...?'

Adopting military sign language, I swept my fingers across my throat.

He wound the window down. 'Is he ...?'

'Dead, mate.'

I'd never seen someone have such a public break down before, but that's what Nigel did. He screamed and cried for England. Perhaps I should have been more sympathetic, but since he'd ignored my pleas to help Lee, *fuck* him.

We drove twenty miles to Castelo Branco, Nigel stopping the car every fifteen minutes to roll a huge joint while still bawling his eyes out. The town had a one-way system and we found ourselves driving around the same surroundings for an hour. It was extremely hot, stressful and confusing, but fortunately an off-duty cop spotted our plight and instructed us to follow him.

I sat in the cop shop still tripping *bombs*. An Arabic-design rug lay on the floor and I watched as it mutated into all sorts of random colours and patterns. On the wall a poster of a woman's head and shoulders warned about the dangers of drink-driving. One side of her face remained unblemished and attractive, while the other half was horrifically scarred. The poster next to it highlighted the hidden harm of domestic violence and featured another female face, only this time it had been beaten out of all proportion. The women's fearful eyes pierced me like black lasers, their damaged features morphing between hideous and grotesque.

Thanks for that ...

Although hallucinating worse than Timothy Leary inside a kaleidoscope I remained calm and collected and able to keep it real. I kept my statement short, explaining how Lee had a couple of beers and drowned. Despite Portugal's progressive drug laws I didn't want to risk being slung into a cockroach-infested slammer. Plus I didn't know for certain what Lee had taken – the post mortem could work that out.

An extremely understanding local man with a connection to the British Consulate appeared and acted as our chaperone. We waited outside the morgue for hours before finally getting the chance to pay our respects to our mate.

It wasn't pretty.

The autopsy had taken place already and the fat black two-inch-long stiches they'd sewn the top of Lee's skull back on with was reminiscent of Frankenstein's monster, his torso crisscrossed in the same crude manner.

Our guide took Nige and I to a plush hotel with much-welcomed air-conditioning. We went straight to the bar and began chain-drinking ice-cold beer. That evening the phone next to Nigel's bed rang, the receptionist informing him it was a call from England. We hadn't been able to contact Lee's long-since divorced parents, having never met them. Nige suggested trying to get hold of Lee's sister, but searching through his Facebook friends list proved futile. As for Lee's mobile it was anyone's guess where that had ended up.

Unbeknown to us the British Consulate *had* managed to contact the family. Yet they'd only told Lee's mother, stepdad and sister 'something' had happened in Portugal.

Nigel stared at me ...

We shook our heads ...

He picked up the receiver.

I'll never forget that scream.

Nige and I parted company in the days that followed. As I placed my backpack on the scales at Madrid Airport the checking-in guy held his hand up, indicating I wait while he took a phone call. Having put the receiver down he frowned and shook his head. The flight in front of mine had just crashed on take-off and one hundred and sixty-seven people lay dead amongst the burning wreckage littering the runway.

Poor people ...

Thinking about those awful phone calls about to take place, I shouldered my rucksack and went to find a hotel. Life certainly seemed precious, making me all the more determined to continue living mine to the full.

Death in Antarctica

You learn more from failure than watching
Coronation Street.

Pablo Picasso

B ack in England life continued to throw up challenges. Mum was struck down with a mystery illness. At first the doctors thought it might be secondary tumours from the breast cancer she'd been treated for a year ago, but having ruled this out they then considered pneumonia. Eventually we were called into a specialist's office to be told she had asbestos poisoning, 'mesothelioma', and three months to live. It turned out Mum had inhaled these tiny yet lethal manmade fibres while working as a nurse in Charing Cross Hospital in the sixties, the place full of asbestos as a result of reconstruction after the war.

Having graduated with a degree in youth and community work only to find there were no jobs, I signed up for a master's in social work. I'd been a support worker in learning disabilities for the last six years for a company called Balleron Care based in Exeter. When my university placement supervisor learned I hadn't received any training, bar one afternoon, from Balleron and only an hour of supervision – both required by law – he shook his head in disbelief and explained that the company were reneging on their duty of care to both me and the clients.

One Friday I finished lectures and got in the car to go and

see Mum. My mobile rang, a manager from Balleron asking me if I could do a sickness-cover shift with a young man I was unfamiliar with. I should have told them a firm, 'No,' but being a loyal nobhead who in six years had never let the company down, I drove to the chap's house. Not long after my arrival he got angry with me over a historic incident I couldn't possibly have known about.

'Don't be so *silly,'* I replied, not giving it another thought.

The other support worker on duty reported me to head office and five minutes later a manager phoned to tell me I was suspended. I didn't think anything of it, figuring I could easily explain the situation, only the company hit me with a disciplinary hearing. I told them there was no malice intended, that it was a light-hearted albeit unprofessional remark. I pointed out I hadn't had any training in my six otherwise-unblemished years of working for the company, never phoning in sick or declining a cover shift, and was under stress from my university demands and my mother's terminal illness – something they would have known about had I received the mandatory supervision.

They fired me for *gross* misconduct!

It didn't end there.

The university ejected me from the master's course, saying I had to take my former employers to tribunal to prove my innocence. Mum beat the odds and lived for a year – the last six months of which I spent researching the law and putting together my own legal case, time I should have been with her. I defended myself against my former employers' expensive lawyer, explaining to the adjudicator how I'd lost my university bursary, a year's salary and a guaranteed job with the city council, leaving me sixty thousand pounds out of pocket.

I won my claim for unfair dismissal ... and was awarded a

measly *four* grand.

And the brown shoes at the university still kicked me off the course.

Oh well!

No one ever said life is fair – and why should it be?

Mum suffered a protracted and painful death, but she did so with dignity and never complained once. When I drove to Cornwall the next day to meet with the undertakers a huge rainbow had sprung up over her house.

Nice one, Mum.

I smiled and have done ever since.

Having scattered our mother's ashes at her favourite walking spot I went home and put the computer on. Rather than curse my former employers I'd use the meagre compensation to keep me afloat while I finished the Hong Kong memoir I'd been tinkering with for years. I decided at that moment to become a bestselling author – so I wouldn't have to work for fucking imbeciles ever again. Only having a GCSE in English and no creative writing experience was irrelevant. The important thing was to take action and ignore the naysayers – and there's always *plenty* of them.

When three years later as an internationally bestselling author I walked through Heathrow Airport en route to my Hong Kong book launch, I smiled to see *Eating Smoke* high in the charts in WH Smith, alongside James Cordon and Gary Neville. Upon arrival in the former British colony I was treated to VIP treatment in the bookshops, an appearance on Radio Television Hong Kong, a double-page spread in the South China Morning Post and hordes of fans at my book signings ...

But there was one person missing from the celebrations.

I'd called Vance Lee, my former business partner, a few years back to apologise for my behaviour when I became so ill from addiction that he had to ask me to leave his flat. 'Ah, *no* problem, Chris!' he'd replied. 'The bissniss go very well at the moment. When you come back to Hong Kong, I make you *manager!*'

I'd smiled, knowing he too was beaming down the line.

Although only a phone call it was one of the best moments in my life. I loved Vance like a hero big brother. That he'd not only forgiven me – or understood how unwell I had been – *and* was offering me a job, spoke volumes about our unique cross-cultural bond.

Eating Smoke had taken me almost two years to write and edit and my Chinese brother had been at the forefront of my mind on every single one of those days, especially after I received a phone call from Blacksmith Books in Hong Kong requesting the rights to publish *Eating Smoke* worldwide and inviting me to attend an official Asian launch.

Having bought an airline ticket I called Vance's office to surprise him with the news we'd be reunited in two days time. To say I was excited to see him again would be an understatement – our reunion was worth way more to me than the book itself.

A secretary answered.

'Lay ho (You good)?' I greeted her.

'Ho (Good).' She replied.

'Can I speak to Mister Lee, please?'

'No ... *cannot.*'

'Oh, why?'

'Mister Lee *dead.*'

'Wha ...?'

'Last month. He die of *heart attack.*'

My ten years of 'all-good character-building stuff' didn't end there. I got a job as a substance misuse specialist for a charity based in Cornwall. Much of my work centred on child protection and involved multi-agency working with a team of associated professionals. I received no end of praise from the social worker in charge for my in-depth knowledge of addiction and above-and-beyond efforts to keep these disadvantaged families together. I put in a whole load of extra hours supporting one particular client, getting her to understand the importance of attending our treatment sessions, thus demonstrating a commitment to the welfare of her three neglected children.

The sticking point was the father, who hadn't engaged with his own drug worker or attended any of the child protection proceedings. This was equally the incompetent worker's fault for not managing his case load appropriately. It got to the point where the children had suffered enough and the social worker would soon have to make the decision to ask the courts to remove them. I was gutted. I didn't want those kids to become separated from their parents and end up in the care system, a sure sign they would suffer the effects of trauma for the rest of their lives.

By pure happenstance I saw the father in passing one afternoon. Knowing the guy was only days away from never seeing his children again, I stressed the importance of turning up to our 'core-group' meetings and the next session with his drug worker.

The father shook my hand, burst into tears and said how grateful he was I'd gone the extra mile to keep him in the picture, agreeing to engage with the process forthwith. But when he mentioned our meeting to *his* substance misuse specialist during their first session together in over *two* years, that colleague reported me to our manager for 'breaking confidentiality'. It was absolute bullshit and a complete misinterpretation of child-protection protocol on the worker's part. Both parents are entitled to know the information exchanged within a core group and every letter of policy backed up my child-centred actions.

Once again I found myself suspended for gross misconduct – only this time I got legal representation and nailed the company for a significant amount of compensation in an out-of-court settlement.

Then with a smile I resigned from the highest paid job I'd ever had.

It was one of the best decisions I've ever made. Life is too short to spend time in a toxic environment and build other people's dreams.

Now that I'd become a published author the only item left to tick on my bucket list was a trip to Antarctica. Then I could kick back and relax for the rest of my life knowing I'd achieved every single one of my life's goals across eighty countries on all seven continents. Perhaps I'd take up knitting or have a go at ballet?

I set about finding an expedition ship to sail to the Southern Polar Circle. My interest piqued when I discovered one of these former Soviet icebreakers offered the option of joining their scuba-diving team. I booked my passage and set about training to the standard required to keep me and my future dive buddy safe in the continent's potentially deadly sub-zero waters.

Having spent a small fortune on equipment and a PADI drysuit course, I found myself diving on wrecks *ten* miles offshore in Plymouth ... *in* winter ... *in* the pitch black. Then

I flew to Bueno Aires and from there to Ushuaia in Tierra del Fuego, the southern tip of Argentina, to meet the expedition ship *Tersius*. It was an incredible experience to sail out into the Drake Passage, pods of humpbacks breeching around the ship and icebergs the size of small countries floating by.

Our utopia wasn't to last …

Tersius anchored off Deception Island and the scuba team clambered into Zodiac speedboats in preparation for our first foray. I'd buddied up with a highly likeable Aussie and fellow international adventurer named Matt. Upon arrival at the dive site Matt and I began shouldering our ridiculously cumbersome equipment and going through final safety checks. Sat across from us in the rubber inflatable were a middle-aged Japanese man and woman. I was amazed at how quickly these two kitted up and rolled backwards off the small boat.

A minute or so later the Japanese pair broke the surface and immediately grabbed the bow rope. The woman appeared to have an issue with her buoyancy control and I vaguely remember Hank, our coxswain and dive supervisor, handing her extra lead weights.

As Matt and I were calmly busying ourselves for our own dip into unknown territory, the culmination of months of expensive training, I didn't pay the Japanese duo too much attention. This wasn't a dive for novices, where you'd expect to see people attaching equipment incorrectly or displaying poor technique in the water. Nor was it a holiday 'fun dive' like in the Tropics, conditions in which you can get away with wearing a pair of shorts and using basic apparatus.

This was a serious underwater excursion requiring complex equipment in freezing conditions in a part of the world so far away from civilisation that no helicopter is going to come and rescue you and no hyperbaric chamber is available should you make a critical error.

In addition drysuit diving comes with a unique set of life-threatening complications and you must know how to rectify them swiftly while keeping a cool head. To dive in Antarctica you're required to have a minimum of thirty hours operational time in a drysuit in a cold water environment and your logbook and certification is checked at the start of the expedition. Therefore you naturally assume each team member can take care of themselves and their buddy.

This wasn't to be the case.

An English woman in *Barbie-pink* diving gear popped up, *feet* first, twenty metres away. Panicking she grabbed hold of her partner, an experienced American diver named Jay. Jay kept telling Barbie that so long as she kept the regulator, the 'air', in her mouth she would be fine, but being face down in the water was giving the woman the impression she was drowning.

It was pathetic. There was no way this amateur had undergone the requisite training required by the expedition.

The dive master put the boat's engine in reverse and began skimming backwards towards the pair – *while* the Japanese couple were still holding onto the dinghy. Having never dived from a rigid inflatable boat, or 'RIB', before, I could only assume this was some sort of textbook rescue drill. But when I looked down at the Japanese girl the ice-cold water was surfing over her face and she had no alternative but to let go of the boat.

Seconds later her buddy did likewise.

Assuming the couple would simply reunite and commence their dive, I turned my attention to helping the pink idiot clamber into the inflatable, agreeing Jay would join Matt and me to form a dive trio.

Matt, Jay and I high-fived and rolled backwards into the freezing blue deep. Sinking slowly to the ocean floor was a momentous experience. I watched in amazement as penguins shot past us and a leopard seal came up to investigate, delighted my expensive Swedish 'Waterproof' drysuit was protecting me from the elements.

Ten minutes into the dive Jay tapped me on the shoulder and made the 'listen' sign. I could hear the sound of the Zodiac's engine revving – the signal for emergency – and so made an immediate controlled ascent.

Matt clung to the rubber boat with a desperate look in his eye.

I had no idea what had happened and so hauled myself with help into the Zodiac to join the rest of the team.

'Matt, what's going on, dude?'

Matt thrust a finger at the Japanese guy. 'His *partner's* gone missing!'

As I sat there trying to figure out what the fuck was happening a second RIB pulled up and we were ordered to climb aboard. The coxswain had already dropped his dive crew back to the ship and was ferrying us likewise.

It wasn't until we were climbing the ship's gangway that everything suddenly made sense. The Japanese diver obviously lacked the experience to maintain a proper position in the water and the extra weight handed to her was probably the *last* thing she needed. When the woman let go of the boat she must have sunk like a proverbial stone and not had the regulator in her mouth. Instead of ditching her weight belt and calmly resurfacing, she must have panicked and sucked in water.

Being a trained rescue diver I felt angry and frustrated. We shouldn't have been pulled from the water – we weren't novices. With the obvious sickly-pink exception all of us were competent divers and members of a team. We should have begun a systematic search – even if it meant snorkelling on the surface (the crystal-clear water was only a few metres deep). By sending the divers back to *Tersius* the ship's crew had unwittingly signed the girl's death warrant.

Our dive team stood at the top of the gangway staring out over the water to the lone RIB. It was twenty minutes before two of the ship's official divers had kitted up and begun motoring out to the girl's last known location. It was *so* stupid. One of the rescue divers was a twenty-year-old biology student. No disrespect whatsoever meant to this young woman, but they'd just extracted a former commando trained as a rescue diver, as well as Steve, a highly accomplished deep-water cave diver, and Jay, who had hundreds of dive hours under his belt, and Lyle, a guy that owned a fucking *scuba shop!*

As the inflatable shot off to the dive site some of the team muttered such naiveties as, 'I hope she's gonna be alright.'

'You better brace yourselves, folks.' I said quietly. 'She's been underwater for forty minutes.'

Fortunately they were able to recover the woman's body, the ship's company and explorers sharing a stunned reality. Not only was it a tragic turn of events but the captain now had to liaise with the coastguard and coroner in Ushuaia to see if the expedition had to be cancelled. Obviously the wishes of the poor girl's family were a priority and no one would have objected to the ship turning about to initiate her repatriation – but that's not to say cutting people's life-long and expensive dream short wouldn't have been an enormous disappointment.

The girl's family requested the expedition continue and

her body was placed in a cold storage room specifically set aside for this purpose.

The next day the dive guides gathered us, the now nine-person dive team, in our briefing room. 'Listen folks,' said Keith, a pleasant and unassuming chap from the Midlands. 'We understand this has been terribly upsetting, so get all the gear packed away and we'll sign you up for some land-based explorations.'

Philip, the world's foremost adventure artist, a solidly built and staunch Irishman who'd joined the expedition so he could paint icebergs *underwater,* raised his hand. 'We came here to *dive,'* he stated firmly.

'Accidents happen,' I added.

'Oh ...' Steve's mouth fell open. 'We assumed you wouldn't want to go back down.'

We were all experienced divers and confident in each other's abilities, which was a good thing too because on the next dive the mouthpiece on my regulator shattered due to the cold and I found myself breathing in icy seawater – *twenty* metres down! By staying calm, having my equipment in order and carrying out the correct drills, I was able to avert a second fatality.

Of course we wanted to get back in the water. Life's for living and that's that.

Ultramarathon Man

Get comfortable with uncertainty, minimise the risk.

Lt. Col. George Armstrong Custer

By the time 2014 scrolled around my life had levelled off somewhat and people stopped dying left, right and centre. The highlight of my year was now an annual trip to the mountains with a large group of snowboarding friends. I still partied at every opportunity and drank my fair share of beer ... but all this was about to change.

My gorgeous girlfriend of three years Jenny came by my house one afternoon in a break between her youth work appointments. 'I'm pregnant,' she announced.

Bummer!

I wondered who the lucky guy was.

Apparently it was ... *me*.

On the running front I'd always kept my hand in, nothing obsessive, just the odd half-marathon, the finishing time of which got progressively slower as my fortieth birthday came and went. 2hrs 5mins my stopwatch once read as I crossed the line three stone over my fighting weight.

In 2010 as I lined up on Plymouth's famous and picturesque Hoe ready for the annual reminder I wasn't as young as I used to be, I spotted my next-door neighbour Daz, a serving Royal Marine. Daz had entered the upcoming *Marathon des Sables,* a gruelling week-long run across the Sahara Desert.

'Hello, mate.' I grinned. 'I could have given you a lift down.'

Our street was six miles away.

'No need,' Daz replied. 'I ran.'

This was my first real insight into serious endurance running. Namely that knocking off thirty-two miles (Daz's total by the end of the day) was something of a breeze for these well-adjusted athletes.

I expected Daz to dash off, but in a display of true Royal Marines' loyalty he dragged me around the course in 1hr 55mins. It was an immensely painful experience, but my brother-from-another had got me back under the two-hour mark and I felt fired up for bigger things.

A kick-boxer mate Jim sent me a Facebook 'suggestion' that I might like an athlete named Dean Karnazes.

What gives?

I clicked the link.

I was met by a banner photo of a bare-chested macho man sporting a pair of shorts and trainers, a focused look in his eye as he ran along a mountain trail. It was taken from the cover of a book titled *Ultramarathon Man – Confessions of an All-night Runner.*

What the hell was an *ultramarathon?* Surely a marathon represented the limit of human endurance? I wasn't aware of anyone on the planet attempting such long-distance idiocy. 'Just got back from a 26.2 mile run through the forest ...' Dean's latest Facebook post read. 'Now I'm off to do the school run.'

What ...? The guy's run a marathon *before* breakfast! What about *recovery* time? What about having quad muscles like *lead* and calves as painful as the *Spanish Inquisition?*

I clicked the 'like' button and surfed to Amazon to grab a copy of Dean's book. Whether consciously or subconsciously my mind was already investing in the future. If runners were putting themselves up for such crazy challenges as going *beyond* marathon distance, then one day I would do the same.

As a result of my never-ending quest for learning I'd begun to see a pattern in the attitudes of life's achievers. Most people who arrive at some form of success start from humble beginnings laden with self-doubt. The thing that sets them apart is they take *action*. Tony Robbins the world-famous personal development guru arrived home one day from his job as a janitor to find a repossession notice pinned to his door. Fed up with life conspiring against him he kicked off his shoes and set off running along the beach. Tony didn't know why – only that if he didn't take *action* nothing would change.

Dean Karnazes had a similar epiphany. This led to him completing the Western States 100-Miles Endurance Race, a circa-thirty-hour trek through the snow-capped mountains and stiflingly hot canyons of the Sierra Nevada, *eleven* times. But before all this Dean was a rising star in a major health-care company. Disillusioned with the American Dream, he realised life in a suit came at the expense of finding the *real* him. Whilst in a bar celebrating his thirtieth birthday Dean put down his beer, turned to his friends and said, 'I'm off!'

'Where?' his surprised crew asked.

'To run thirty miles.'

'You're crazy!' they replied to a person.

'I might be crazy,' said Dean. 'But I'll be a crazy person who's run thirty miles.'

And the rest is history ... and a *damn* good book.

I moved in with Jenny in preparation for our new arrival,

temporary name 'Junior'. Personally I hoped for a girl, so 'Junior' was interchanged for 'Martha' every so often. Jenny's house was in the city centre, which opened up a load of new running routes for me. With the ultramarathon phenomenon on the backburner in my never-say-never mind, I began increasing the distances and got a buzz from the sport like never before.

Often I'd set a 5am alarm and go for a jog under the sodium-yellow glow of streetlights through a deserted Plymouth and the historic Barbican port, stopping to photograph fishing boats chugging out into the jet-black Sound. Running across the Hoe's mile-long parade at sunrise was a real Rocky Balboa moment – minus the pint of raw eggs and getting my head punched in. On Sunday mornings I'd run past packed-out pubs, feeling unusually removed from the drunken debauchery spilling out under a cloud of nicotine onto the pavement.

Soon I was easily knocking off half-marathon distances, carrying my bankcard so I could stop at service stations to buy a bottle of water. I downloaded the Endomondo app onto my phone and invested in a heartrate monitor. Seeing distances go up and heartbeats come down provided a real incentive to keep pushing out the miles three times a week.

On weekends I upped the distance, heading down a section of the National Cycle Network, which ran through a forest and followed the disused Great Western Railway tracks and a fast-flowing river. Then I'd cut across Dartmoor before re-entering Plymouth's urban grey sprawl. Thirty-something miles was the most I managed but it took me to the limit of my physical fitness, legs seizing in pain, leaving me in serious doubt of completing a decent-sized ultramarathon.

'Martha' popped out and decided to be a 'Harry'. Jenny

and I couldn't wait to get out of the hospital with our bundle of ... *boy.* We ran for the door as soon as the discharge papers had been signed – and I hardly slowed down when we got home.

'You okay with Martha ... *erh,* Junior ... *erh,* Haz, for a while?' I asked my number one girl.

'Go!' She smiled.

I put my headphones on and ran a marathon.

As I sat at my desk working on the second book, *The Trade,* in my Hans Larsson thriller series a thought popped into my mind, *Why don't I run the length of the UK, from John O'Groats to Land's End?*

The idea of packing camping gear into a rucksack and taking a jog down the spine of Britain struck me. I began to envisage the idyllic locations I could pitch my tent in at the end of the day as veggie sausages sizzled in a pan over an open fire. Moreover I visualised the 'me' time I'd have to reflect on life. By then Haz would be one year old, but Jen wouldn't have an issue with my plan. That's the wonderful thing about waiting for the perfect partner to come along. They believe in *you,* so you don't need permission to live your dreams in order to grow as a person.

After a two-minute discussion with my girl I booked a flight to John O'Groats from Exeter at the end of the summer, then bought an ultralightweight tent for the snip of £500 and a 300-gram Mammut sleeping bag for £400 on eBay.

My training began paying off and I was able to run the Torbay Half Marathon in one hour fifty, my fastest time in twenty years.

Quite often I found myself thinking back to my London Marathon, when thirty metres past the finish line I'd sat down against some railings to recover and spend a moment celebrating my personal victory. The chap getting his breath back next to me said he was a 'double Ironman'.

A double ironman?

I'd been extremely impressed by the idea of a five-mile swim, a two-hundred-mile bike ride followed by *two* marathons and had made a mental note to one day compete in such an event – although you can safely exchange 'compete' for 'complete' in my bucket-list approach to life.

With this particular dream simmering on the backburner I started going to Plymouth's Life Centre to improve my swimming. In my first session I managed fifty metres, forced to stop and cling to the side to recover. But an ironman was my goal and my heart would see it through.

An advertisement for a twenty-four-hour race run in five-mile laps in the grounds of a majestic stately home in the Cotswolds popped up on my Facebook page. Seeing how *far* I could run in a day appealed to me. Surely I could beat my thirty-two-mile personal best?

I had a problem though. Whilst running a half-marathon around my regular seafront route I'd experienced pain in my right ankle. Having kicked off my brand-new Karrimors, I found I'd worn right through the rubber tread on the outside of both heels and my right peroneal tendon was once again 'clicking', an injury I hadn't had to endure since going alkaline.

On my bookshelf was *Born to Run* by Christopher McDougall, an international bestseller and quite possibly the most authentic and organic account of running ever written. For some reason I'd not read my copy since buying it on Amazon two years previous. I had a vague idea it was a book about 'form' as opposed to Dean Karnazes' somewhat more heroic account of the sport.

I settled down with a cup of tea to read it.

In a quest to rid himself of perpetual pain resulting from his favourite pastime Chris journeys to the Copper Canyons in Mexico to track down the Tarahumara, a reclusive Indian tribe rumoured to cover enormous distances on foot. Clad in simple sandals fashioned from discarded car tyres the Tarahumara enjoy a pre-fifty-mile-run breakfast consisting of corn beer, joints of weed and a simple porridge. Chris asserts the reason the Tarahumara never get injured is due to their natural 'forefoot' strike, whereas westerners have been hoodwinked into landing on our heels by the eighties' explosion of spongey running shoes. The author kicked off his trainers and immediately cured himself of 'plantar fasciitis', a condition that had plagued him for months.

Armed with this information I booked an appointment with the physiotherapist and embarked on my first shoeless run – across three miles of the Dartmoor National Park. To say the experience felt amazing would be an understatement. There's something incredibly natural, *primal,* about running as nature intended. It adds a whole new interpretation to the sport, one I would never have believed possible. I hopped over muddy puddles, skipped gazelle-like around patches of spiky gorse and shortened my stride to negotiate other obstacles – such as the liberal sprinkling of landmines of the pony and sheep variety. Not once did I worry about stepping on anything sharp, glass or thorns for example. My eyes naturally honed in on these potential dangers and I avoided them with ease.

The big day – or should I say 'weekend' – arrived. On the Friday night my brother Ben and I drove to the Cotswolds and pitched our tents in the stately home's majestic grounds.

When I lined up for the off at 9am the next morning, sports tracker on my phone switched on, MP3 player charged and a bag of vegan pasties and a bottle of rum stashed under a tree, I had no preconceived race plan. My sole concern was whether or not my ankle would hold out. As a precautionary measure I'd strapped up the injury using stretch tape. When the starter waved us off I concentrated on striking on my forefoot and a maintaining relaxed upright posture.

Surrounding me were entrants of all size, shape and ability, from serious players to fun runners, some competing in a team relay. The former all appeared to wear the right kit – brightly coloured trail shoes and a jazzy-looking waistcoat with built-in water bladder and umbilical drinking hose, plus mesh pockets to hold energy drinks, snacks and gels.

I settled into a leisurely pace, essentially a jog, mimicking the guy to my left, who I chatted to for the first lap. We approached a grassy hill and I readied my athletically-honed mind for the charge up it … surprised when my temporary running partner slowed to a *walk?*

I'd read something about this, the all-important technique distinguishing ultra-distancers from say marathoners. It's the same concept employed by soldiers on speed marches – walk uphill and run the downhills and flat. This is why ultrarunners are able to cover such vast distances. It also explained why I'd never managed more than thirty-something miles before, not without my legs seizing up and head feeling like death.

Another important tactic is to never let yourself get out of breath. While trotting along, chatting and power-walking the steep parts, I began to understand how our persistence-hunting ancestors were able to chase down large game over enormous distances, as detailed in *Born to Run*.

The race was a delight to compete in, the course

meandering through forests, fields and up the main drag of the stately home, taking in a mile of country lane for good measure. Halfway into the five-mile lap a refreshment stand offered all sorts of goodies, the appetite for each treat differing as the day wore on. Chocolate-coated roasted coffee beans, for example, would have made me feel sick at 10am, but come two in the morning I'd be scoffing handfuls of them as if my race depended on it. Jelly babies seemed a popular choice as did plain old drinking water in the heat of the summer. For me though, the high point of the day was brewing up a pint of Yorkshire tea on my multi-fuel stove – and splicing it with rum of course.

The homemade vegan pasties went down a treat and were pretty much all I ate on the course. I stayed away from energy drinks and sickly snacks, worried I might get a deceptive sugar rush for half an hour and then suffer a crash – although at three-thirty in the morning it feels great to shovel anything calorific into your mouth and you don't seem to notice any mental or physical peaks and troughs.

The afternoon threw up my only challenge.

Ouch!

An intense pain shot through the ball of my right foot. I pulled off the shoe expecting to find a thorn or perhaps a nail penetrating the sole ... only there was *nothing*. Attempting to complete another lap I was in too much pain to continue and sank down on the edge of the track to massage my foot.

'You alright, bud?'

I looked up to see a fellow runner.

'Chris.' I shoved my hand out.

'Mike,' said Mike, shaking my paw.

Mike Brewer was a serving Army officer and a genuinely kind man. He helped me hobble back to the start line, where upon closer inspection it appeared I had a corn or similar under the skin. Just touching it brought back the shooting pain.

'It's gotta come out.' I shook my head and asked Ben to run back to the tent and grab my Swiss Army Knife.

As Mike went to fetch his first aid kit I dug the scalpel-like blade into the offending spot and carved out a knot of flesh, leaving a gouge the size of a pea. Mike then bandaged my foot and we were off, the pain from the wound insignificant when compared to before.

Come 7pm I'd completed my second marathon, walking part of the last lap with a chap who'd swapped his trainers for hiking boots and a set of walking poles. I admired his ingenuity, but this method looked a truckload of hassle and I was happy to simply plod on. I stopped by the tent to brew another cuppa, amazed I'd run over fifty miles and didn't feel even the slightest bit fatigued.

By three in the morning, twenty more miles in the bag, my legs felt stiff – but to put things in perspective I'd suffered five times as much whilst running half marathons. I was chuffed to bits my ankle hadn't given me any grief. I'd bashed out seventy-odd miles and it was the easiest event I'd ever participated in. I was glad I'd brought a powerpack so I could top up my phone on the hoof – this way I didn't lose track of any mileage on my Endomondo app.

As I hadn't set myself a goal – bar enjoyment – I decided to call it a night and continue after some food and sleep. I returned to the tent and cooked up a pan of soup, veggie sausages and beans. Washing my well-earned feast down with yet another cuppa was heaven as far as I was concerned. I set my alarm for 7.30am and enjoyed a three-hour nap, then slipped my trainers on and headed back to the start line.

I caught up with Mike halfway around. He'd done an all-nighter, an all-out attempt to get a hundred miles in the bag. I admired his determination.

A young woman appeared on the horizon. She looked *out* of it – red-faced, sweating and exhausted in the extreme. I assumed she was cracking the big 'one hundred' too.

'You okay?' I tendered.

'*No ... no,*' she gasped. 'This is the *hardest* thing I've ever done.'

'You've got that right,' I fibbed. 'What lap are you on?'

Mike was on lap fourteen and me thirteen, so I expected to hear similar.

'My *first,*' she wheezed. 'I'm in a relay team, but they can get *lost* if they think I'm doing any more!'

We pulled alongside a chap who'd stopped to walk up the lane. Gavin Boyter was an affable Scottish chap and a writer and film director. Like Mike, Gavin had done the non-stop thing, despite having a historic knee injury giving him grief.

'I should probably have quit,' panted Gavin. 'But I'm running the length of the UK soon to make a film.'

'Wow, I'm doing that too,' I told him. 'But I don't envy you carrying all that film equipment.'

'I'll have a support team,' Gavin puffed. 'Staying in hotels as we go.'

'Gotcha.'

Mike and I crossed the line together and swapped contact details. Then this generous-hearted soldier suggested we stop by the officials' tent to check the race results.

Mike had run seventy-eight miles. This surprised me because I'd slept for three hours and still knocked up seventy-six – according to my tracker. Gavin had done amazingly well with 101 miles, but the top competitor Paul Beechey managed an astonishing 123.

I drove back to Plymouth glowing with an enormous sense of satisfaction. I'd proved to myself that covering long distances held no problem – indeed, it was far easier than running shorter ones. And my ankle had held up. Now I had the length of Britain to look forward to next summer and the time to get some training in.

Barefoot

If in doubt, shake it all about.

Stephen Hawking

I went to see Ken, the physio at my GP centre, to get treatment for my clicking ankle.

'Reverse strain exercises,' he said, cutting a metre-length of rubber strip from an industrial-sized roll. 'You've got to work the tendon in the opposite direction to what it's used to.'

Back home I looped the rubber band around a leg of the sofa, hitched it around my toes and did the stretch for twenty repetitions, but after several weeks it still hadn't made any difference. By now I was hooked on barefoot running and had familiarised myself with the leading proponents of the sport. I read books and watched videos by such zany individuals as Barefoot Ted and Barefoot Ken-Bob, guys who easily ran marathons on Mother Nature's tyres. I began to visualise running the length of the country shoeless.

My first run after the twenty-four-hour race was a jog around the local park. Only, as opposed to the other runners wearing expensive running shoes and clutching fist-held water bottles like adult dummies, I had on shorts, a heartrate monitor and *wetsuit* boots. The booties were an experiment into running without the usual cushioned soles. They worked well for this three-miler, although my feet began to squelch towards the end.

Linked to the Endomondo app on my phone the heartrate

monitor told me my pulse while exercising and how long I spent in the rest, aerobic and anaerobic zone. In the past I'd once had a resting heartrate of fifty-three beats per minute, down from eighty, and I wondered if I could ever get back to this level of fitness.

I bought a copy of Scott Jurek's *Eat and Run,* not knowing this book would have a huge impact on my life. Scott is one of the world's top ultrarunners, having won the Badwater Ultramarathon through Death Valley twice and the Western States 100-Mile Endurance Run a record seven times. Even more fascinating is that Scott only eats plants, dispelling the myths around humans depending upon meat as a source of protein. I'd already significantly reduced the amount of factory farmed flesh in my diet and Scott's example made me more determined to continue on this path.

To save money I became a member of the Life Centre. Membership included access to the gym and sauna, the latter being one of my favourite pastimes. I was amazed at how difficult learning to swim front crawl proved to be but clung to the advice that it's all about technique. I did enjoy the swimming though as well as the progress I was slowly making having watched endless YouTube videos. I increased my two lengths to ten and managed to get the time for them down from ten minutes to seven, bringing me closer to my goal of ironman. The biggest surprise however came in the gym. I found I struggled to do one pull-up, the twenty-nine I'd managed in my Royal Marines days now a distant memory.

The Life Centre offered the use of a local athletic club's running track, so I stopped off twice a week after work for a four-miler. The drawback with the barefoot approach is your feet need time to adapt to not wearing shoes. All the literature advises the newbie to take things steady for the first couple of years, but *Surely injury won't happen to me.*

I bathed my feet in surgical spirit but it didn't make any difference and when I upped my speed on the track the soles burned and blistered. The pain from a partially prolapsed disc also increased, a problem that had initiated during my time in the military. I bought a pair of gravity boots online so I could hang upside down from the pull-up bars in the gym, hoping this extreme form of stretching would rescue my worsening condition.

While running barefoot around the park I decided to venture onto the road and ended up completing a seven-mile circuit of the city. Treading on paving slabs and smooth tarmac proved no problem – but the rougher surfaces resulted in agony beyond belief. When friends heard about my newfound passion their reactions sadly leapt to the negative – as if I'd announced a plan to barbeque hedgehogs as opposed to getting in touch with my physical, spiritual and human self. 'What if you step in dog shit?' was the most asked banalitism.

'Why would I want to do that?' I'd reply.

My boss wasn't happy with my request to take six weeks unpaid leave the following summer to complete my JOGLE. But if she didn't give me the time off I'd resign. Life's not about conforming to other people's pension plans and preventing someone achieving their dreams falls nothing short of slavery.

I conducted several more seven-milers barefoot around the city, but rather than hardening up the soles of my size sevens became increasingly sensitive. Along with the soreness the balls of my feet developed hard elliptical sacks of fluid under the skin, known as a bursitis. I had no idea of how long they lasted – it certainly didn't seem as if they were going away anytime soon. Little did I know they weren't to be my biggest problem.

On Gavin Boyter's Facebook page I could see he'd blitzed through Scotland and most of England and had now entered Devon. I arranged to meet him en route. Gavin was pleased I'd made the effort and flicked on his GoPro to film our five miles together. It was great to listen to Gavin's story. I was surprised to learn he'd worn the same pair of trainers all the way from John O'Groats. I couldn't see that being the case for me – not with my John Wayne gait.

We stopped for lunch with Gavin's support crew – which at this point in time consisted of his delightful mum and dad, who both seemed surprised I'd be embarking on my length of Britain run solo *and* unsupported *and* sleeping by the side of the road.

October 2015 was upon us and the Great West Run was upon me. A mile from the half marathon's finishing line I was on for an improved time, somewhere around one hour forty-eight, but instead of charging home I pulled over to the side of the course, removed my trainers and socks and shoved them into the waistband of my tracksters.

I couldn't have picked a rougher surface on which to go barefoot. It was *agony* – but I couldn't show this to the cheering crowd. Still it was a great feeling to experience the thrill of going shoeless in a major race and running on the smooth white line proved to be my saving grace.

Whether I'd run my JOGLE barefoot remained to be seen, but at least my fitness was on the up. Albeit expensive I had bought the two most important parts of my equipment – my tent and sleeping bag – and I knew I could run up to seventy-six miles each day and still have time to sleep. I took a week off work with the intention of undertaking a practice run from Plymouth along the Coastal Path to Land's End.

On the Friday afternoon before my departure on the Monday, I set off for a gentle four-miler in trainers. I was happy and had a plan.

What could possibly go wrong?

Tested

Ahhhh!'
I broke into a walk on Embankment Road, which runs alongside the River Plym estuary. The dodgy disc in my spine had finally collapsed. I limped two miles home in pain beyond belief and crawled into bed still clad in my running gear.

'You okay?' asked Jenny.

'No ...' I grimaced. 'I'll have to cancel my coastal path run and spend my week of leave in bed.'

My spine was so damaged badly that a week turned into three. The only time I got out of bed was to visit the GP surgery. The doctor I saw practiced being useless. In so much pain I couldn't even sit in the chair, opting to kneel on his office floor to relieve the pressure on my sciatic nerve.

Rather than recognise I needed immediate surgery he sent me away with ... *co-codamol.* The pills were so useless I had to wash double the dose down with a can of beer every morning just so I could change position under the covers.

When I finally went back to work my supervisor Paul called me over. I assumed he wanted to welcome me back and check I was okay.

'We're putting you on an improvement plan,' he announced. 'If you take any more time off, we'll issue you with a warning for misconduct.'

'*Misconduct?* Paul, I couldn't *walk!*'

'If you're not capable of doing your job then it's a disciplinary matter.'

There was nothing I could say or do. It was typical of the modern workplace. It simply made me more determined to sack off this dead-end employment nonsense at the first opportunity.

I attended an appointment for an ultrasound on my ankle, only the nurse in the radiology department said my GP should have requested an MRI. I then saw a specialist who put me through such a brutal range of lower-limb exercises – *'MORE! MORE! HARDER! HARDER!'* – that I wasn't sure if the guy was a sadist or I'd wandered into the recruiting office for the Navy SEALs by mistake.

When my feet finally came to rest he frowned. 'You've got extremely high arches.'

Was this good, bad or freakish?

'It means you naturally over-pronate. Oh, and your clicking ankle is not severe enough for surgery.'

'But it's severe enough for me, Doc,' I replied, realising the consultant was penny pinching on behalf of the NHS.

All a keyhole surgeon had to do was grind a slightly deeper channel in the ankle bone to prevent the tendon from slipping over it every time I took a stride.

'When I do my length of Britain run it's bound to get worse!'

'Then I'll recommend your GP prescribes you painkillers.'

My dodgy disc relapsed to the point where I had to take more time off work. Figuring swimming fixes everything I limped to the pool, pleased I could now complete 250 metres in under six minutes. It didn't help my back though and I found myself on another prescription of co-codamol.

My dad kept reminding me a chiropractor had fixed his slipped disc with a 'gentle nudge' and so I made a reluctant decision to visit one. This 'adjustment' malarkey sounded utter quackery, unsupported by science or logic.

By the time my appointment at the plush practice in Plymouth arrived I was in more pain than words could capture. I now spent all day in bed – on my side, top leg crooked to relieve the pressure on the nerve. I swear I'd rather have summited Everest naked than cram myself into a car to go and see a back doctor. I couldn't put my seat belt on in Jenny's Toyota as I had to crouch in the footwell.

Getting out of the car was the worst fun I'd ever had. So too was limping across the car park and *lying* on the waiting room floor. Not even my gorgeous little boy lighting up the other patients' faces could bring a smile to my own. To make matters worse the guy I saw was an Aussie. Don't get me wrong – Aussies are fine if you need someone to drink a swimming pool full of beer or beat up a crocodile, but letting one of them attempt to fix your spinal column so he can fund another trip to Amsters is a step too far.

I warned the quack my back was really bad, but the scammer insisted on dropping what felt like kettlebells on my lower vertebrae.

'You've made it *worse,* Doc,' I hissed.

'Nah. I can't make it worse, mate,' he scoffed.

The fucking idiot had and the agony was now too much to bear.

Rather than forward me for an immediate MRI scan and emergency surgery my moron of a GP reluctantly upped my dose of painkillers to include tramadol, which accomplished nothing. I stayed awake all night howling like a soldier shot on the battlefield. All Jen could do was to hold my hand and tell me it was going to be alright.

It was far from it and in the morning I begged her to call 999.

The paramedic could only give me air.

I already had air – shitloads of the bloody stuff.

I crouched in the footwell of the ambulance car as he drove *flat out* to A&E ... where I then waited three hours to be seen.

A medic approached and gave me an ultimatum. I could either wait for a bed or get a 5ml dose of Oramorph to take home with me. I was so desperate for pain relief I accepted the latter.

'Excuse me, sir!' asked a stunned nurse moments later. 'Why are you *crawling* across the car park?'

'My cab's arriving and I can't walk.'

'Wait, I'll get you a wheelchair.'

'But I can't get *into* a wheelchair.'

'Oh ...'

Jen had to call both 999 and 111 in the week that followed. On the second occasion, a no-nonsense German doctor arrived at our house, gobsmacked to learn my GP had refused to issue me with proper pain medication.

'But you're a forty-seven-year-old *adult!*' she fumed. 'What does your GP expect you to do – stay in bed the rest of your life?'

This Teutonic angel wrote to my doctor telling him she was placing me on a prescription of Oxynorm, a potent liquid form of synthetic opiate, and for the first time in months I was able to get out of bed and not have to pee in a bucket.

I finally had an MRI scan and went to meet a spinal surgeon in Salisbury's private New Hall Hospital as there were no NHS ones operating in Plymouth at the time. Within seconds he ascertained I needed a 'discectomy' – although I had to wait a further six months on top of the year I'd already spent disabled.

I'd been planning on having a year off alcohol for longer than I cared to remember, having started drinking at thirteen, when I'd neck pints of my old man's 9% homebrew.

In the forces I'd always drunk to excess on a night out, as is the norm, and had enjoyed some brilliant experiences – as well as numerous mishaps. I'd loved drinking beer whilst out travelling the world, not to mention that alcohol had seen me through some extremely tough times, eradicating the pain of loss, rejection and an at-times solitary existence.

A can or two of beer in the evening had also helped me kick my amphetamine habit, but more recently the negative effects of this slow and socially accepted killer had started to outweigh the positives. Now that I was a father it was important to set a balanced example for Harry.

As is often the case with breaking bad habits I first needed a wake-up call. Mine came at 4am on a bench in London's Paddington Station. I'd travelled to the Smoke for a military reunion but had got so pissed on the early evening train I must have sat down in the station to check my accommodation details and fallen asleep. Fortunately my daypack was still tucked under my arm and no harm was done, but this didn't mean it was appropriate behaviour for a guy with a loving partner and child who depended on him. It was the final straw and I decided to have a year off the poison.

My twelve months without beer proved so worthwhile that when the anniversary of my sobriety came around I decided to continue. By now I'd had my spine operation but the opiate medication was proving problematic. There was no denying I'd needed powerful meds to kill the extreme agony. However, the price you pay for taking such high doses of a super-strength drug is physical and mental dependence, culminating in an enormously painful struggle to get off the bloody stuff.

At 4am each morning the hideous withdrawal symptoms would begin – akin to the infamous scene in *Trainspotting* – and I'd reach for the first of my four daily fixes. Within seconds sheer bliss would initiate as if a troop of massaging angels had lifted my angst-laden body into the clouds to chill out to Goa trance with God.

Groundhog Day continued and the months flew by as my routine of balancing the highs and lows and a career and family rolled into one. Fortunately I had the self-awareness to initiate a strict reduction regime, during which I entered a period of self-growth, studying anything that promised to usher me further along the path of enlightenment. When my best friend Simon drank himself to death it bolstered my commitment to mastering my emotions and living the *pura vida*.

But there was something else. I'd been on the medication for such a long time that I think the biochemistry in my brain had changed. What I'd been mistaking for withdrawal symptoms was in large part due to a condition named PAWS – Post-Acute Withdrawal Syndrome – which meant even months after getting off the Oxynorm I continued to experience a constant ringing in my ears, severe cramps, night sweats and a general feeling of unease.

Let's Do This

Stop talking, start running.

Ant and Dec

Another health issue that came to light as the medication wore off was a severe pain in the right-hand side of my lower back. Somehow the degeneration in my spine had trapped a nerve, which after everything I'd already been through was extremely disappointing. I began hitting the swimming pool at six every morning followed by a sauna and self-referred for physio at Derriford Hospital – but really didn't hold out much hope. I knew I needed a second operation, which according to the surgeon involved bolting the sacroiliac joint in my pelvis together with titanium rods. Beth the physio I saw at the hospital encouraged me to stay positive and the exercises she instructed me in got rid of some of the discomfort.

Following my swimming and gym sessions the ensuing endorphin rush helped to temporarily alleviate the PAWS symptoms. However, every morning come 4am my ears would start ringing, legs in spasm and sweat pouring, meaning I never got enough sleep. I changed my diet to ninety-eight percent plant-based and read up on the age-old practice of water fasting.

Water fasting entails ... *drinking water!* The longer you fast the better the results, with forty days being the generally acknowledged limit. Most people find the idea of going without food abhorrent, but for every human bloodline that exists on this incredible planet the ability to fast has been encoded in its DNA. Our hunter-gatherer ancestors would have gone without food for weeks when faced with times of scarcity and unpredictable environmental conditions. The miracle of evolution has led to the human body integrating these glitches into maintaining the health of our species, so going without food on occasions actually increases vitality and longevity – and not the other way around.

The benefits of fasting verge on miraculous, especially when combined with meditation as many of the ancient Eastern texts espouse. A water fast removes toxic substances, fat and acid from the body and can reverse ailments – including life-threatening ones – that might ordinarily require surgery or long-term medication and which an individual may have suffered for years. By decalcifying the pineal gland or 'third eye' a fast enables your mental computer to access and neutralise deep levels of filed trauma, the likes of which other therapies cannot reach.

By day three of my fast I no longer thought about food. By day ten I entered a beautiful state of being as close to mental freedom and understanding as I reckon it's possible to get. Niggling issues that had bubbled under the surface for decades, ones no doubt driving my addiction and other impulsive behaviour, floated out of my head like helium balloons and disappeared into a brilliant blue sky. I felt utterly amazing, three stops past incredible, like raving in Ibiza with Fern Britton and an expense account. When after eighteen days I went back to eating, I knew I could go out into the world and smash it.

I knew I could achieve *anything*.

Now I was off the meds, eating a plant-based diet and suffering a lot less pain my thoughts returned to running the length of the UK. I couldn't live knowing I hadn't nailed a dream goal. Having contacted my surgeon and explained the situation I requested an emergency procedure – anything that would enable me to set forth from John O'Groats.

Back I went to hospital for what must have been the twentieth time for an exploratory injection into one of the nerves in my spine. Paul my surgeon needed to ascertain the pain was coming from my sacroiliac joint and not the lower back. He told me he would inject a third dose of steroids into the area in an attempt to pinpoint the problem.

While mentally mapping out my upcoming challenge I spoke to Baz Gray, a former regimental sergeant major in the Royal Marines and a mountain-and-arctic-warfare specialist. Baz had so many awe-inspiring accolades under his belt and had raised thousands for the Royal Marines Charity. He'd run 189 miles nonstop and taken part in an expedition to recreate Shackleton's epic escape from Antarctica. His current plan involved skiing to the South Pole in what would likely be the harshest conditions to date for such an undertaking. A man to be respected, Baz told me in no uncertain terms that a JOGLE attempt would be foolish with my health problems and I'd be better off focusing on recovery.

My book cover designer, former marine Andy Screen felt likewise. 'You're mad. High-performance athletes can't run a thousand miles nonstop, let alone someone with a crumbling spine.'

I fully respected my brothers' looking out for my welfare but I still had to complete the JOGLE at some point. You only get one life – so it wasn't as if I could postpone it until the next one.

I travelled up to Salisbury for my spinal procedure, which appeared to eliminate much of the pain. As such I booked a new flight to John O'Groats for August 31st 2018. This meant if I could run the length of the country in three weeks I'd be home for my 49th birthday. The big off was only a month away and so at least I could get some training in.

I coughed ... and coughed again.

Before long I was hacking like a fifty-a-day smoker.

I'm not sure what was up. I'd been to visit my GP months ago because of strange viral-like symptoms I'd been experiencing. The blood tests I had done all showed me to be perfectly healthy. Perhaps withdrawal off the opiate medication had something to do with this persistent shallow cough. Or maybe it was because I'd continued to exercise and sauna whilst on the water fast – something you're not supposed to do – and this had depleted my system of vital nutrients. Whatever it was it couldn't have been worse timing, what with my run only four short weeks away.

I'd love to have done at least a *wee* bit of training before my 999-mile JOGLE – especially as I'd been disabled for over two years. I mean who the hell tries to run the length of the UK unsupported without *any* preparation whatsoever? But all the sports literature I'd read over the years stressed the importance of not exercising when your body's fighting illness. In addition the latest spinal procedure hadn't worked, which confirmed the damage lay in the sacroiliac joint.

Oh well! I crossed my fingers and started getting my equipment together.

K.I.T – three letters that strike more fear into the heart of an ultrarunner than a rattlesnake in a phone box. I'd always adopted a straightforward approach to the subject – no Vaseline, tape, energy gels or 'Gucci' CamelBak bladders, just a reasonably priced pair of trainers and the promise of some water somewhere on the course.

For the JOGLE I figured I'd take my regular camping gear and stove plus a waterproof jacket for when it rained and a fleece for the night time. I reckoned what with the lightweight Nordisk tent and a set of custom-made carbon-fibre poles I'd bought, along with my thermals, roll mat and sleeping bag, the weight would be around five kilos.

How *wrong* could I be!

If you're planning to walk a thousand miles then the 'eighteen kilos' my bare minimum of kit totalled would present little problem. But for running, especially with my broken back, it was recipe for the hospital. I *had* to get the weight down.

I'd learned in the marines that having a properly fitting rucksack or 'bergen' is crucial when load carrying. If the bag is too short the waist strap rides up under the ribcage, putting unreasonable strain on the shoulders and spine. I had a well-fitting twenty-year-old Lowe Alpine bergen – only it weighed *three* kilos. So rather than fork out £300 for a lighter pack I decided to jettison some fabric. Every night for a week I sat in the front room, scalpel, scissors and sewing kit to hand, discussing my journey with Jenny whilst hacking off unnecessary pouches, straps, webbing and zips. I ended up with a backpack half its original weight.

My kit still totalled over sixteen kilograms, before food and water, so I threw caution to the wind and began replacing it with the lightest gear available. I swapped my bulky North Face fleece for an ultra-high-tech Haglöfs hoodie and bought a gas cooker the size of my thumb. A foil wind shield for the stove weighed less than a Bic biro and – *Phew!* – arrived from China the day before my departure. As far as training shoes were concerned, rather than experiment with the increasingly popular and generously cushioned 'Hoka' brand, I decided to buy another pair of Karrimor waterproof trail shoes, the ones I'd worn without problem in the twenty-four-hour race.

Baz my former-Royal Marines regimental sergeant major buddy called. Baz was a director for the Baton foundation, a not-for-profit military charity staffed entirely by volunteers. What with all my injuries and lack of training I'd been tempted to disappear off to John O'Groats in secret, but it would have been insanity not to raise funds for veterans in a similarly traumatic situation to the one I'd found myself in all those years ago. As such I decided to run in aid of the Baton and welcomed Baz's expert expedition advice.

Upon hearing my bootneck mind was made up, Baz switched into military mode. 'Right, comfort is important if you're running up to fifty miles a day ....' he said, beginning a conversation that encouraged me no end.

When I mentioned the mysterious virus-like symptoms and unshakeable cough I'd been plagued with for months, Baz said, 'Just get on the road, Chris. What's the worst that can happen?'

I phoned my designer Andy Screen to ask if he would sponsor me by knocking up a banner photo for my #999miles social media pages. 'No problem, Chris,' he replied without hesitation. 'And if an ultramarathon is any distance longer than a marathon, then why not promote "An ultramarathon a day for 999 miles?"'

'Good thinking, mate,' I told him – although neither of us were factoring in the fourteen-kilo bergen weighing heavily on my shoulders.

A week before my flight the pain in my sacroiliac joint became unbearable. Obviously I didn't have time to go getting my pelvis bolted together and so I pleaded with my surgeon for a last-minute nerve-numbing injection. 'Can you make it to Salisbury tomorrow?' Paul asked.

'I'll be there,' I replied.

'You really ought to have a practice training run and camp out,' said Jenny. 'To test your kit.'

In an ideal world my thoughtful partner was right but I still had this weird virus and cough and was desperate to recuperate. I resolved to spending the next five nights under canvas in the back garden instead. The one-man Nordisk tent proved immediately problematic, its cramped interior a haven for condensation, which drenched the down-filled bag and left me shivering in the early hours.

Each night, I experimented with differing combinations of thermal underwear, sleeping systems and ventilation, all resulting in me becoming wet and cold. Worse still the temperature in Plymouth was four to six degrees warmer than the Scottish Highlands. With this in mind I made a last-minute trip to Go Outdoors, where the understanding manager kindly sold me a three-seasons bag at their staff's discounted price. I hoped this would put an end to my sleeping issues.

I'd spent countless hours getting everything together but still hadn't planned a route. Yet there was a reason I'd paid scant attention to maps and coordinates. I wanted to show my young followers on social media the importance of ignoring the naysayers and escaping our wrapped-in-cotton-wool culture. If you over-plan an adventure your mind conjures up imaginary obstacles and you can end up talking yourself out of your own dream. Besides, I was travelling to John O'Groats not the Mongolian Steppe and so long as I had a south-pointing compass, telephone and my bankcard what more planning was there?

By now I'd spent over two-thousand pounds on equipment and flights – not to mention what would eventually total several weeks of lost income. With sponsorship in mind I approached Marc Spender, an unbelievably generous former army chap I'd met through my writing. The director of an online business, 'I'm *in!*' Marc replied and bunged me five hundred quid.

Mark Beresford, a former marine and Falklands War veteran, ran a company called Bootneck Money. Another of the most generous men I've ever met, 'Put me down for five hundred' he said after our three-minute exchange.

Following only two hours' sleep I was still working on my kit and an MP3 playlist the morning of the flight from Exeter Airport. *Fourteen* kilos my pack weighed – and this was with the bare minimum of food and no water in my military-issue army-surplus-bought bladder.

I thought about my clicking ankle ... my year-long virus-like symptoms ... my prolapsed disc and busted sacroiliac joint ... the brain damage from the opiate medication ... the unpleasant sweats and spasms I suffered every night ... the ZERO training I had done ... the ridiculous weight in my bergen ... the growing group of supporters on social media ... the HUGE military support building ... all the people who would expect me to fail ... the press and media attention ... the mental health community that I *couldn't* let down ...

If I had been in good health with a truckload of training under my belt, if my backpack weighed a modest four kilos instead of fourteen, I'd be ready for the challenge ...

Only ... I *wasn't* ready, *was* I.

As anxiety consumed me I turned to my amazing girlfriend and whispered, 'What am I *doing,* hun?'

'You'll do it, Chris ...' She chuckled. 'You *always* do.'

'Yeah, I *will.'* I grinned. 'I'll *fucking* smash it!'

Paul Basford

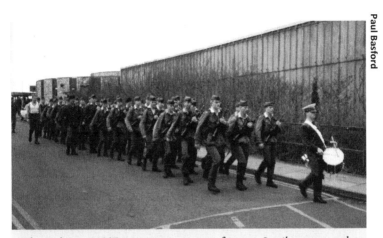

The Fighting 558 Troop entering camp after our 9-miler commando test. I'm seventh back on this side – not the position I ran in!

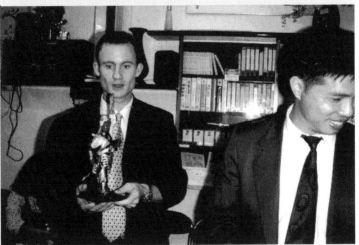

With my Chinese brother and business partner 'Vance' Lee Hok Keung (R.I.P) in our office in Hong Kong.

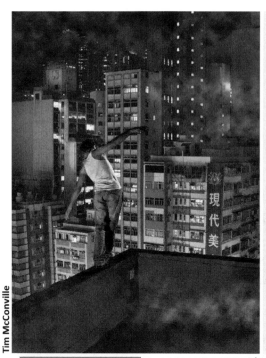

Tim McConville

The cover image for the Hong Kong edition of *Eating Smoke* – pretty much sums up my experience over there.

A kind solicitor represented me free of charge. '... a severe psychiatric illness ... the prognosis is poor.'

Dear Sirs,

Christopher John Thrall ▮ **Carroll Road Crownleaze Plymouth** ▮
Roll No. ▮

We act on behalf of the attorneys of Christopher Thrall of ▮ ▮ Devon.

Mr Thrall is regrettably suffering from a severe psychiatric illness. At present, the prognosis is poor. There are no assets, he has no earnings or means of satisfying any debts due to him and we are in the process of registering his enduring power of attorney. A copy of a short medical report is attached.

It is unlikely that he will ever be in a position to clear any debts.

As to the final prognosis, it is not thought that any firm indication will be possible until a period of approximately 3 months. Can we suggest therefore that you put a moratorium on any debts owed by Mr Thrall. The matter can be reviewed at the end of 3 months, by which time there may be some more information, although as we have said the initial medical opinions are that it is going to be some years before Mr Thrall is better.

Yours faithfully

▮ & ▮

106

My firewalk to raise money to study as a development instructor in post-war Mozambique.

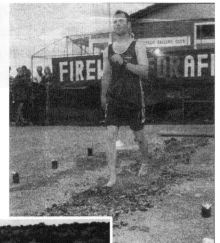

Plymouth Herald

Fishing with the street kids I taught in Africa.

Driving volunteer journalists to India and back by coach. Lee (R.I.P) and I breaking the 'rules' as usual, enjoying a beer on the Turkey/Iran border.

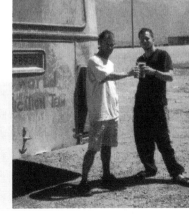

The London Marathon 2005 – as you can see, I'm in the lead.

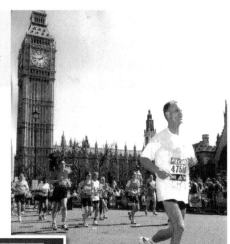

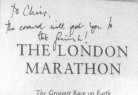

To Chris,
the crowd will get you to
the finish!

THE LONDON
MARATHON

The Greatest Race on Earth

John Bryant

My copy of *The London Marathon* signed by the author. 'The crowd will get you to the finish' – yes, John, plus the 26.2 miles I have to run!

Certificate

This is to certify that

CHRIS THRALL

Runner number 47558

Successfully completed the Flora London Marathon
on the 17th April 2005

The Official Finishing Time was

03:56:30

Overall Finish Position: 9651 out of 35105
Mens Finish Position 8139 out of 24641

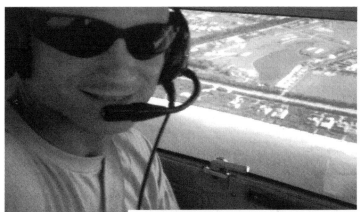

Getting my pilot licence and AFF skydiving qualification in Florida – slightly warmer than scuba diving with icebergs while on an expedition to the Antarctic Polar Circle.

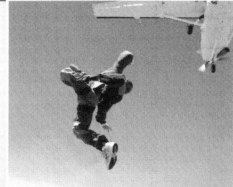

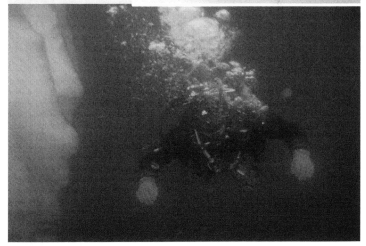

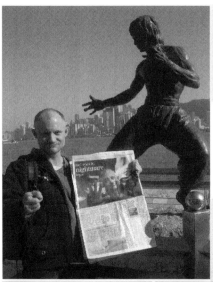

With Hong Kong's #1 son on my return to Hong Kong to launch *Eating Smoke*. Choose your role models wisely!

Running 76 miles in the Cotswolds 24-hour race. I was surprised at how easy it was.

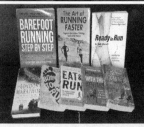

To become a better runner, I read several books – and thoroughly enjoyed them.

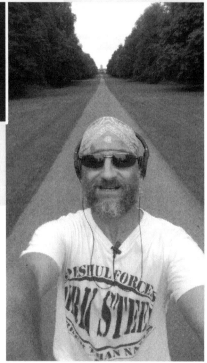

John O'Groats

*It's not the getting knocked down, it's whether you can
laugh while you're down there.*

Obi Wan Kenobi

Day 1 | John O'Groats to Wick | 20.44 Miles

John O'Groats, how breathtakingly beautiful, how *remote!*
Having checked out of my glamping pod
accommodation at 11am I stood beneath the famous white
metal sign post, comforted in the knowledge it was only 3,147
miles if I needed to swim to New York. A vast lavender-grey
cloud bank stretched overhead, beneath it a thin strip of pale
blue rescuing the otherwise gloomy day.

It was a later start than anticipated as I'd been up since six
with a needle and thread reattaching the straps on my bergen
as they needed to be two centimetres higher. Load carrying is
an art and you intuitively know when your set-up is right.
Even then you'll still adjust the shoulder and waist straps up
to fifty times a day, redistributing the pack's weight to relieve
an aching neck and hips.

Alan Rowe, founder of the Baton charity, had phoned to
introduce himself during my stopover at Edinburgh Airport –
or it might have been Glasgow. Seriously, this wasn't a
sightseeing tour of Great Britain. I was here to run #999miles
to Land's End in the fastest time possible and so long as my
compass pointed south I wasn't concerned with place names
or historical locations. A kind and humble man, Alan

extended me the charity's full support, explaining how as a barber for over half a century he'd cut the hair of thousands of military personnel, many of whom's histories dated back to the Great War. I'd ended our call knowing I wouldn't let him – *or* our veterans – down.

It was hard to believe the donations on my Virgin Giving page totalled £600 already. I gave a Facebook video update to my growing number of supporters, explaining who I was and what I was doing, urging folks to at least share my posts if they couldn't afford to chuck a fiver in the pot. Then I started running to Land's End – or home as I thought of it, Devon being the adjacent county to Cornwall.

I didn't run very far – quarter of a mile back to the Seaview Hotel. The previous evening I'd filmed a muster of my kit, thinking some of my followers might be interested, but after an hour logged onto the hotel bar's Wi-Fi the video still hadn't uploaded, so I downed my lime and soda and got on the road ... and it was *absolutely* brilliant!

The rain held off and the sun burst through the forbidding black curtain, enhancing the beauty of the purple carpet of heather lying all around. I knew the upcoming A9 would prove a road safety nightmare, but jogging along the near-barren B-road out of John O'Groats I experienced utter bliss, despite my knees going through a range of pain and the bergen torturing me with all fifteen of its kilos.

I found myself thinking of a game plan for the voyage ahead. Obviously due to my lunchtime start this would be a twelve-hour day, so I needed to run half an ultramarathon. However, I didn't want to get all uptight about the mileage thing. This once-in-a-lifetime pilgrimage had cost me and Jenny thousands of pounds and if I found an idyllic spot in which to pitch camp and absorb the nature, one that happened to fall just short of ultramarathon distance, I wanted to take full advantage of it. The same went for stopovers that made sense practically or for issues of safety – suitable ground to plant the tent or near a water tap or shop. With this in mind I resolved to 'average' an ultramarathon a day over the course of the trip and not take a day off until I reached Land's End.

It was tempting to reflect on the enormity of the task in hand, but I *stamped* on those thoughts there and then. I was running to Land's End and averaging an ultramarathon a day – *end of!* There was *no* other option. There's nothing to be gained by contemplating 'what ifs' and potential obstacles and hardship. I was doing this thing – even if I had to crawl all the way – and would live in the moment and appreciate it. The only future image in my mind was seeing my Jenny and Harry at Land's End when I smashed this challenge out of the park.

I ran along listening to my MP3 player, songs I'd heard a thousand times before but which sounded so much more energising and uplifting now. Spoilt by the stunning seascape and rolling heathland and stress free for the first time in months, I was in heaven. Then my phone rang, interrupting sheer bliss and the *Rocky* soundtrack.

'*Thrall,* you always were a *crazy* fucker!'

It was Jock Hutchison, my troop commander from Royal Marines training.

'*You* can talk, Boss!'

'*Hah!*'

It was great to catch up after thirty years and realise how much this endeavour meant to folks. Jock invited me to his ranch in Inverness, offering to lay on a big welcome with press, media and so forth, but this posed my first dilemma. How could I accommodate these kind offers without compromising my ultramarathon a day goal?

Another issue bound to come up was food. Moreover bacon butties. My Royal Marines family would no doubt wish to support me all they could, but this would likely result in a well-intentioned conveyor belt of bread-and-pig slices – a bootneck staple – and I wanted to stay as close as was practical to a plant-based intake due to the physical performance and mental utopia an alkaline diet produces. I didn't want to snub kind and generous offers though and the occasional bit of meat would be fine.

I continued down the A99, the luxury precursor to the juggernaut-laden A9, heading to the airport town of Wick, approximately twenty miles away. In the cab the previous day I'd pictured myself running back along this road. The feeling it invoked is hard to explain – a mix of real and surreal, my mind wary of the large number of sharp blind bends. I passed several hamlets, some made up of ancient stone buildings, others clusters of latter-day bungalows. Each village had a roadside cemetery filled with gravestones ranging from simple slate markers to miniature mausoleums atop with Mother Marys and angels.

As I perused the names of the dead whilst questioning the sense of misery and loss aroused by this somewhat peculiar age-old practice it began to rain, forcing me to cover my shirtless torso with the ultralight Haglöfs jacket. I didn't bother wearing a t-shirt or my faithful running smock underneath as they would only become soaked with sweat in minutes and I had no means to dry them – other than inside my sleeping bag at night, only adding to the dampness in the tent.

Just as I was wondering if Hamish McDonald had died in *every* village on my route, two fellow enders approached from the south, 'ender' being JOGLE/LELOG slang for pilgrims travelling from one end of the country to the other. Both of these chaps had backpacks and hiking poles and one was tethered to a Jack Russell.

'Guys!'

We shook hands and I learned that Mike the dog owner had walked the length of the UK over the course of two years during his holidays. The other chap Ed had completed the route in three months. Ed had slept in a tent and it was interesting to note he'd averaged fourteen miles a day carrying a similar weight to mine. Ed gave me a heads-up for a Weatherspoon's and camping spot in Wick. He also recommended the West Highland Way, stressing its rugged beauty and conveniently distanced backpacker hostels. I congratulated the boys on only having twelve miles to go and we said goodbye.

I had no fixed plan for today. Despite months of inactivity and my lack of training, the running proved no problem – it's a state of mind. My knees were going through some pain though. I kept forcing myself to slow down but the awesome tunes and stunning vista soon sped me back up again. So long as I had water to rehydrate it didn't matter where I stopped. Wick offered a park to sleep in along with a cheap pub breakfast and free Wi-Fi for a Facebook update and twenty-two miles seemed a sensible distance for this first 'half' day.

After eighteen miles I started to feel the effects of jogging all afternoon carrying so many kilos on an empty stomach. Some noodles would go down well and a cup of Rosy likewise and so I sat on my backpack in the gateway to a field to get the cooking pot on. I was happy with my progress and delighted by the initial experience, but most of all I was pleased about my killer mindset. The scenery was gorgeous, the running out of this world, yet all of this took second place to hugging my girl and little boy at Land's End – *job done!*

Approaching the outskirts of Wick I began looking for a place to lay my head for the night. I stopped to check out a derelict house. Crashing on my inflatable mattress on the bare concrete floor would save me the hassle of packing the tent away in the morning and give me a bit of elbow room to boot. All the windows were boarded up and so I explored the eerie rooms with my head torch on, finding the whole place covered in a thick layer of bat shit. The deciding factor was water – or the lack of it. I had less than half a litre and the resultant dehydration during the night would trigger my brain damage and initiate those hideous leg spasms.

I continued onwards and within a few hundred yards found a café. It was shut but the outside toilet had been left open. I checked the water was from the mains and not a roof-top holding tank – a distinct possibility in these remote parts – and added a litre and a half to my water bladder. As a litre of water weighs a kilo such considerations were important. I contemplated returning to the deserted house but, as in life, we *never* go backwards, we *only* go forwards.

A Tesco superstore sat on the edge of town. I spent an inordinate amount of time choosing a small chopping board and a Tupperware box to hold perishable items of food. Then I bought some bananas, plus an onion, leek and broccoli to spice up and alkalize my next noodle fix. On a salt craving I grabbed a tin of anchovy-stuffed olives.

It felt strange to walk into Spoons wearing my running gear and backpack on a drunken Saturday night. I ordered a lime and soda and veggie bangers and mash and settled at a table in the corner to upload the kit muster video to Facebook. This wasted two hours due to the pub's weak Wi-Fi and so I made a mental note to stick with live streams.

I left the bar at 11pm, found the park and began setting the tent up in an area I deemed clear of canine land mines and away from interfering eyes –

Blue lights erupted on the nearby road ...

A cop car *screeched* to a halt ...

Two young male bobbies wearing stab vests and wielding heavy duty Maglites *charged* across the grass ...

'Good evening, officers!' I grinned, attempting to deescalate any potential problems with some 'please don't put me in jail' politeness.

'You!' the nearest bobby yelled.

Oh fuck ...

'You're the one we saw *running* from John O'Groats!'

'Hah!'

As I explained my mission to highlight veteran suicide to these kind and appreciative officers, I knew I'd secured a safe sleeping spot – but since when did they let thirteen-year-olds join the Old Bill?

Day 2 | Wick to Forse | 17.97 Miles

'Ah-ah-ah-ah-ah!'

Bloody seagulls!

I checked my G-Shock – 4am – *damn!* I'd hoped what with the previous day's exertions for a decent night's sleep, only the birds had triggered the ringing in my head and three and a half hours would have to do.

The gulls weren't my only problem though. The amount of H2O in the cramped compartment, a combination of rain, breath and sweat, had led to a remake of *Waterworld,* and the three-inch-deep puddle on top of the sagging flysheet hadn't helped. As a trained commando I could handle a bit of cold and damp, but in the Highlands a wet down sleeping bag could lead to life-threatening hypothermia. Because I needed to get on the road I didn't have time to wait for a spot of sunshine to dry everything out.

After a cuppa and token wet-wipe bath I packed up and made my way to the pub, pleased my legs weren't *too* sore. While waiting for a breakfast of toast, tomatoes and mushrooms I strung the tent across two chairs and headed to the gents. But when I arrived back at the table – *Nooooo!* – my bum-bag had *gone!* Luckily I'd had the foresight to shove the phone in my pocket, but what about the MP3 player, sunglasses and compass? Although futile I began checking through the rucksack – *Phew!* – and found the handy holdall tucked under the top flap. What an *idiot!*

By the time I'd eaten and posted to Facebook it was approaching 11am. *Where the hell did three hours go?* To keep my ultramarathon-a-day dream alive I'd have to seriously speed up these refreshment stops, limiting them to the time it took to fast-charge my mobile on the triple USB plug I'd invested in. The expensive power bank I'd bought as a back-up source was both heavy and a waste of money. Once its juice had depleted I would never have three hours spare to recharge it. I had additional music and audio books and podcasts stored on the phone, but not wishing to drain its precious battery and risk interrupting the tracker, I'd stuck to listening to my MP3 player – although the hundred and fifty or so tracks had begun to repeat.

After a check of the charity total – almost a *£1000!* – I kitted up. Leaving Wick the A9 rolled through heathland and golden corn fields, the barren sea appearing magnificent to my left. The road had become 'official', earning itself white lines and a much smoother, liquorice-black surface. Unlike the previous day, during which local motorists knew to give us enders a wide berth, the growing traffic was now a serious consideration and the highway potentially lethal.

In view of the headphones being a permanent fixture on my bonce, I had to reassure one person during a Facebook live update that I didn't have music on. This was a slight white lie as I still listened to my MP3 player through one earpiece. I could never turn the tunes off completely – they were proving to be an enjoyable and highly motivating part of the experience. A couple of folks expressed concern I was running 'with' the traffic, so I explained I had to swap sides every so often otherwise the camber of the road wore the muscles in my right leg out.

Neoprene compression sleeves are supposed to aid circulation in your lower legs and thus reduce inflammation and injury. I'd never worried about this sort of thing before but wore a pair now just to be on the safe side. The weather was glorious, the sun beating down on my shirtless and already-bronzed skin, but what I hadn't bargained on was the river of sweat running down my calves. At first I blamed the waterproof Karrimors for my dripping wet socks and sore toes. It wasn't until I pulled off the road and sat down in a farmer's field to brew up a cuppa that I realised the compression sleeves were the cause of the problem and for the first time ever I had blisters. The fact my feet had swollen a size wasn't helping.

Sitting amongst the stalks of wheat, sipping a cuppa whilst drying my piggies, I spotted a fellow ender heading south in *flip-flops!* Madi was a delightful English woman of Indian descent who I'd met on the plane. She was raising money for a global charity supporting women in impoverished communities to kickstart farming initiatives.

As we walked along the road, chatting and dodging the speeding cars, Madi explained she planned to stay in hotels and have her luggage forwarded by taxi each day. The reason Madi had ditched her walking boots was the enormous blisters on *her* toes, ones she'd lightly bandaged. We worked out my heavy bergen and two late starts were the reason for our tortoise-and-hare scenario.

I'd been putting a lot of thought into the extreme amount of weight on my back. I now had a more informed perspective of the challenge ahead and the vital kit required – as opposed to kitchen-sink luxuries. I made my mind up to find a post office and send some stuff home. If I could lighten the load by a kilo then that would be an awful lot less jarring compression on the body over the course of millions of foot strikes.

After a pleasant half-hour together Madi decided to call it a day and phone a cab, only she didn't have a signal on her mobile so I offered her mine. 'Are you sure?' she asked.

'Of course.'

But as Madi put the phone to her ear she tripped and supermanned forwards, instinctively shoving her hands out – with my Samsung clasped in one of them!

I watched in horror as the poor girl slammed into the tarmac and the phone ground across the rough surface – *screen* facing down.

'Whoa, are you okay?' I helped the girl to her feet.

Madi's hands and carefully bound feet were in bits, blood trickling down her wrists and oozing from her toes. I'd never seen so much claret appear in a relatively minor tumble.

'Your phone!' Madi stared at the damaged screen, mouth agape.

'Forget it. Let's get you sorted.'

I genuinely wasn't bothered about the phone itself – despite it being a pricy S8. There were several chalky white gouges down the screen, but my only concern was whether the technology still worked, namely my comms, tuneage and navigation.

A flick on the ON button confirmed the little fella was still in the land of the living – unlike its predecessor who I'd somehow managed to run over in the car. I called the cab, shoved the mobile back in my bum-bag – or 'gentleman's leisure accoutrement' as I preferred to think of it – and helped clean up Madi's wounds.

Even though I was tired, aching and had covered over thirty miles in under twenty-four hours, I began to run *faster* ... and *faster*. In view of my not training for three years, the pace verged on ridiculous and so I forced myself to slow down for fear of injury.

Arriving in the tiny village of Lybster I was delighted to find a post office but undelighted it had shut. I'd only run thirteen miles today and wasn't sure whether to find somewhere to pitch the tent – the local football pitch looked promising – or continue onwards. I was desperate to lighten my load and didn't want to risk not finding another post office for a day or two.

Upon hearing my predicament the woman in the corner shop immediately offered me her back garden. She added that there was a post office in Dunbeath, seven miles south. Hunger – moreover an energy craving – got the better of me and so I grabbed a loaf of raisin bread, a bag of milk bottle sweets and a ginger cake. Then I thanked her profusely, intending to hit the highway, only I couldn't resist stopping for some proper food at the village's upmarket pub.

After I'd found a seat and ordered 'Skink', a traditional Salmon chowder, two bikers leaned over to ask what I was doing. 'I'm ex-RAF,' one of them announced, pulling out two Jock ten-pound notes and telling me my meal was on him.

As I wolfed the dish down while inspecting my poor suffering feet the air force biker sidled up to my table and whispered, 'The guys at the bar are kicking off, mate, because you've taken your shoes off in the pub.' He winked and patted me on the shoulder.

Fair one, I suppose ...

Having paid my bill I slipped out of the side door.

I intended to reach Dunbeath seven miles away, only it was getting dark. By the time I'd finished telling Harry a bedtime story whilst jogging along, it was pitch black. I considered putting on my red-flashing LED safety lights. However although travelling fast the traffic was sporadic and I couldn't be arsed to stop and take my rucksack off. In fairness I'd managed almost fifty years without getting knocked down and had no intention of starting now.

The rain soaked me to the skin in seconds and reluctantly I began searching for a camping place. All the land around these parts appeared to be smallholdings though and I didn't want my headtorch attracting the unwanted attention of Farmer McGiles. The verge was too overgrown to pitch a tent and so I settled for the corner of a field, hidden from view behind a thick stone wall and huge oak tree. I just had to hope a branch didn't fall on me during the night. Little did I know it's what's known as 'common land' north of the border and you're entitled to camp anywhere.

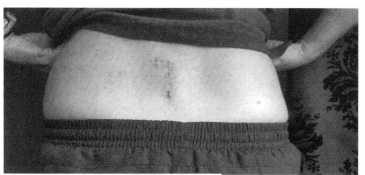

'Ouch!'

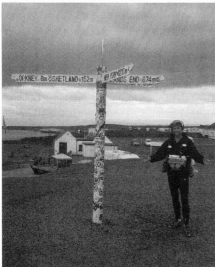

Reality check – one of the two famous signposts. This one is at the start line in John O'Groats.

Compass – 'South' – Let's go!

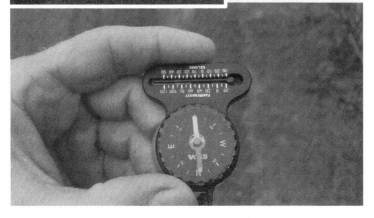

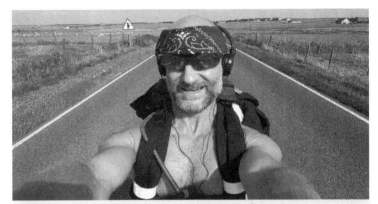

Finally on the road – just BRILLIANT!

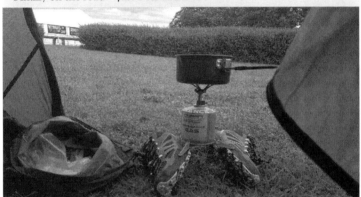

Waking up in the park at Wick.

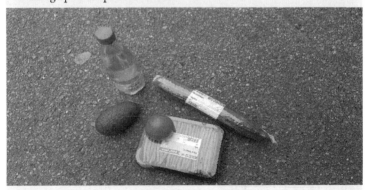

Keep up the greens – staying alkaline.

Broke not Broken

You're never too old to let the miles unfold.

The Milky Bar Kid

Day 3 | Forse to Lothbeg | 29 Miles

'Moooooo!'
Bloody cows!

It was 4am and so I inserted some foam earplugs and snoozed for another two hours. Then I made a cuppa, did the wet-wipe-wash thing, packed up my gear and hit the road. I still felt fighting fit, only my knees were playing up – general pain and nothing specific. As far as the running was concerned it continued to be wonderful fun, particularly as I had a growing group on Facebook posting thoroughly supportive comments.

My followers on social media seemed amazed I was running to Land's End, but not many appeared to comprehend the enormity of my 'personal' challenge – namely averaging an ultramarathon a day carrying a full set of camping equipment and sleeping by the side of the road. One Facebooker even asked me what bike I was riding and another the walking boots I had on my feet!

I ran along as happy as can be, making up alternative names for the places I arrived at. 'Lybster' became 'Lobster' and 'Whaligoe' 'Way to Go!' As for 'Mid Clyth' and 'Occumster' ... let's not go there. Moreover I looked forward to arriving at the post office in Dunbeath to shed some of this surplus kit.

On the edge of the tiny village I stopped for brunch, setting up my cooker on a large flat-topped black rock. 'John O'Groats this way, buddy?' huffed a cycling American ender.

'Yeah, but it's closed today, bro.'

'What!' He slammed on the brakes, staring at me aghast.

'Just kidding!'

After a bowl of veg and noodles I went into the sole shop and asked for the post office.

'Other side of the valley,' said the guy serving, pointing to an *enormous* hill.

This will hurt ...

It didn't though and I ran the mile-long slope with surprising ease. Then after purchasing a large plastic envelope I mustered my kit on the side of the road and adopted a mercenary approach to what stayed and went.

I had eBooks on the phone and so my paperback, *Dark Summit,* could go. Thermal underwear likewise - my tracksters and T-shirt would have to do – a slight gamble what with the Highlands ahead. My running gloves, a precautionary measure, were now history – I'd wrap my hands in my sleeves if necessary. The power bank for the phone went along with four pairs of socks, an expensive set of gel insoles and a few other bits and bobs. With the exception of teabags, powdered milk and two snack bars, I shoved my food reserves in the post office's outside bin. I'd buy more as and when required or go hungry until I found a shop.

In the end the package weighed a kilo and the bergen felt so much lighter, although the increasing pain in my right knee and hips and shoulders more than offset the small gain. Furthermore the cough plaguing me for months had kicked in good style.

I had a Facebook comment from Colin MacLachlan of TV's *SAS: Who Dares Wins* fame saying he would come and meet me when I reached the Forth Bridge. It would have been great publicity for the charity, but the Forth lay to the east of Scotland and I planned on continuing down the west to pay my respects at the Commando Memorial. I would try and accommodate people's kind offers where possible, but it was important to stick to my own plan and run #999miles and not 1200.

My phone rang, Steve Sellman, an old buddy of mine from recruit training. 'Mate, it's amazing what you're doing. You can count me in for an anonymous five-hundred quid if you make it.'

I was blown away by Steve's generosity, but the 'if you make it' was redundant from my perspective. I *would* make it – simple.

The A9 had become hilly and lethal in places, with no verge on its blind twisting bends. The steep inclines proved no problem though, but I found myself having to sink into the hedgerow and take pot luck with nettles and brambles to avoid the monster-sized trucks thundering past. At the ten-mile point the pain in my right knee had grown almost unbearable. I'd tried using the expensive gel insoles before sending them home only they'd compounded my swollen feet issue. This trip was certainly proving a learning curve. I pushed on nonetheless, determined to complete at least another seventeen miles and crack an ultramarathon.

Having made a promise to attend to my feet the minute they threatened to blister I sat down on the verge next to a thick pine forest to change socks. In an instant thousands of minute flies descended on me, the likes of which I'd never seen before. Bang on cue as I fought to remain calm and address my feet Jenny phoned.

'I'll call you back!' I yelled – multi-tasking not my strongest point.

Running down the road with a rucksack certainly piqued people's interest. When my phone only had twenty percent battery left I stopped at a tearoom to charge it and keep the Endomondo tracker working. Four elderly folks leaving the tearoom engaged me for half an hour about what I was doing and why. It was worth taking the time to speak to members of the Great British public as many of them subsequently messaged me via Facebook to say they'd made a donation to the Baton charity.

I ordered a coffee and the woman in the tearoom started with the 'mocha-locha-chocha-chino' inquisition – when a straightforward mug of Nescafé would have done.

Although it was frustrating having to wait for the phone to charge I passed the time listening to the adventures of a French cyclist. When I finally got back outside I started scanning around for my bike ... before realising with a dose of stupidity that I didn't have one.

As I approached the town of Navidale a recently deceased black-and-white moggy lay in my path, blood dripping from the poor creature's nose. I saw a sign for the Navidale House Hotel and when the proprietor answered the phone I asked if he owned a cat. He said loads of strays hung around the premises and didn't appear too bothered when I informed him there was now one less.

In a newsagent's shop on the high street I bought some much-needed salad.

'Where are you running?' asked the woman behind the counter.

'Land's End.'

'Oh, my *mother* ran around Britain.' She beamed.

'Wow!'

'Then someone beat her record and so she did it again.'

Double wow!

Day 4 | Lothbeg to Brora | 4.89 Miles

'Baaaaaaaah!'

Bloody sheep!

I unzipped the sleeping bag and stretched my aching body, the ringing in my head particularly bad this morning. Although pleased I'd managed twenty-nine miles the previous day, my back was sore, my right knee the embodiment of torture. Worse still I knocked over my tea while brushing out the tent.

Following a wet-wipe bath I got on the road, only it was no good. I couldn't put weight on my knee and had to resort to walking.

Bummer!

It was tempting to regret running an additional twenty miles yesterday on a busted hinge but there were to be no negatives on this trip. I'd smash this JOGLE *somehow*.

After limping for three time-wasting miles I crashed my shirtless self in a field and came up with the newspeak term 'blistified' in a Facebook update. It was heavenly reclining on my backpack in the sun and so I decided to enjoy the moment and risk using the last of my water to make noodle soup.

Then I ran along scanning the houses I passed for an outside tap to fill my water bladder. I felt hesitant to knock on a door. Everyone was so friendly here I kept getting held up in conversation.

Approaching the town of Brora, I saw a sign.

Royal Marine Hotel.
Half a mile on the left.

Brilliant! Right when I needed a bit of TLC an establishment run by one of my brothers-in-arms appears. How *lucky* was I!

I limped onwards, picking up the pace as I couldn't wait to see a member of the 'family'. I could picture the scene – me entering the foyer to see a chunky ruddy-faced bastard looking up with a smile.

'Hello Royal!' I'd greet the balding crusader.

'Brother!' he'd reciprocate and we'd bearhug for Brora. 'Fancy a wet?'

'Fuck it, I'll have a beer!' I'd reply – making an exception to my teetotality for this most special of circumstances.

Yes, I could see it! Before long I'd be ditching my dusty kit in the hotel's honeymoon suite – on the house of course – grabbing a shower to rival the Angel Falls, then hitting the town with my *buddy,* my *bessie,* my *oppo,* before rolling home shitfaced at 3am to crash in satin sheets – *Sweet!*

As I passed a rolling and well-manicured golf links with a stunning sea vista an enormous country house appeared. My brother-from-another was certainly doing well for himself. I entered the lavish reception and approached the reception desk.

'Whey-hey!'

A frail elderly gent turned around, a mix of blank and startled on his gaunt face.

'Royal!' I extended our in-house welcome, thrusting out my palm and figuring the bearhug was in the can and coming to a

cinema near me.

'R-r-*royal* Marine Hotel ... yes.' He offered a feeble handshake and looked as if I'd come to eat his grandchildren.

'You're ... *not* a bootneck?' I continued.

'A boot –?'

'Never mind. This hotel *is* named after the Royal Marines though, right?'

'"Marine" as in sea view, sir.' He pointed out the window. 'And "Royal" because Princess Anne once stayed here ... *and* her dog.'

'Right ...'

I mumbled some nonsense, about-turned and headed for the door.

A green cross appeared and so I popped inside the shop to ask about my painful knee.

'How far have you run?' asked the pharmacist, a professional-presenting middle-aged woman with blonde hair.

'About eighty miles – over three days, that is.'

'What!'

'From John O'Groats,' I clarified, surprised this wasn't obvious. 'On my way to Land's End.'

'Well, *not* anymore.' She shook her head. 'Your knee is severely inflamed and needs at least three weeks rest – *and* ice.'

So that's the official prognosis ... I thought, deciding I didn't hear it.

I could afford to take half a day off and not jeopardise my ultramarathon-a-day average – but simply give up? *Not* a chance, Lance!

I entered the somewhat plush Sutherland Inn and ordered a delicious bowl of cauliflower soup, an enormous salad and a bag of ice from the extremely welcoming young woman behind the bar. Having overheard me explaining my vagabond state to the girl, a wonderful couple Steven and Christine Arnott, touring Scotland in their campervan, paid the bill.

The ice certainly helped but it wasn't enough to get me back on the road and so I treated myself to a load of snacks from the Co-op and set out in search of a place to rest up. A patch of neatly mown grass from which the 'You are entering Brora' sign sprouted would do nicely. I climbed into my sleeping bag and caught up on some much-needed sleep.

That evening I made a live Facebook video update informing my supporters of the pharmacist's insistence I stop, adding I was fine and not going to make any rash decisions overnight. I didn't tell my online companions I had no intention of calling it a day as I didn't want to trivialise the seriousness of the injury, not with the nine-hundred miles that lay ahead.

Day 5 | Brora to Glenmorangie | 27.34 Miles

I woke at 4.30am to an influx of messages and comments, many along the lines of 'Well, you did your best. You can go home now. No shame in that.' Others suggested getting a hotel for a week, going to a GP or finding a hospital.

I understood this advice was well-intentioned, but some individuals were so vocal in their insistence I give up I couldn't help wonder if they wanted me to fail. I was genuinely surprised people thought I would wrap my hand in so easily. Jenny and I had made a significant investment in both time and money, and suicidal veterans – although unbeknown to them – were counting on me. It was an ultramarathon a day average to Land's End and nothing else. I fully respected that walking the length of the nation is an admirable achievement – it's just not what I wanted to achieve.

After packing up I hopped over a hedge into a field to … *check* for crop circles and with a degree of injury fuelled trepidation got on the road.

Fuck!

In the chill of morning my knee hurt more than ever and now my opposite hip was giving me grief. The cold was a significant concern, the elevation only set to increase as I entered the mountains. I found myself ruminating on my decision to send the thermal gear home.

One step at a time, Chrissy …

I already regretted jettisoning my gripping paperback. While lying in the tent yesterday I'd listened to the audio edition of Ant Middleton's *First Man In* instead. Ant had told me he was planning on writing a book and I was thoroughly enjoying it. However, to get me started in the morning it had to be a party prescription of *thumping* tunes – either Abba, Jedward or Jason Donovan's third album. I could listen to Ant's memoir later in the day.

Passing a boarded-up bungalow I clocked an outside tap and stopped to fill my water bladder. The tap hung down from the eaves on a nylon pipe and the thought occurred to me the source might be a rainwater collection tank on the roof. Having learned from my costly mistake in South America that time, I added a couple of sterilisation tablets and after an hour the water was safe to drink and tasted normal.

As clumps of fir trees and deciduous wood began to break up the otherwise barren landscape my phone rang. Alan from the Baton had seen last night's Facebook update and was offering to put any medical, equipment or accommodation needs on his personal credit card.

In Golspie whilst queuing in Mitchell's Chemist to buy a knee support, I considered taking him up on the offer, only with me and Jenny having spent so much money already it felt a bit needy asking for £16.99.

With the neoprene sports bandage wrapped around my leg I ran two-hundred metres and dumped it in a rubbish bin. My knee problem wasn't of a structural nature. It was something else altogether and the sleeve was of no use at all.

I stopped in the Co-op to indulge an old habit – coffee. These days I mostly stuck to tea, far less acidic on the body, but a carton of the Columbian export wouldn't hurt. Besides, a couple of years ago I wouldn't have hesitated to grab a beer for the road and so this minor lifestyle lapse still represented a significant advance.

At the Trentham Hotel pub in Poles I ordered a vegetable curry. It was great being on an 'official' mission. Rather than um and ah over prices on the menu I had a legitimate reason to order whatever I felt like. I still had to pay for it though and estimated my food bill would be over a thousand pounds by the time I reached Cornwall.

'And you're injured *already?*' the beard behind the bar cocked his head.

Jeeze, thanks for that, mate!

His doubting Thomas act was a slight kick in the crotch.

It was becoming apparent that other people's attitudes, particularly on social media, would affect my moral if I didn't take action. This was the pros and cons of opening yourself up and exposing your challenge of a lifetime to public scrutiny – generally great support but interspersed with ill-thought-out comments.

I decided to make a Facebook update to request folks adhere to some mission-friendly and goal-focused ground rules. Once again I reiterated my commitment to arriving at Land's End *without* taking a day off. I explained my posts about injury were solely to make my supporters aware of the level of difficulty involved in running such a distance and not an invitation for them to feel sorry for me. I added that if people continued to try and talk me out of my dream I would just shut up about the aches and pains.

A few followers had written 'You should have done some training!' and it was hard not to feel irked as I'd already explained the reason behind this – namely that I'd been *disabled* for three years. Besides I *was* training, wasn't I? I was running an ultramarathon a day carrying thirteen-plus kilos – you can't train much harder than that!

I closed my video update by saying there wouldn't be any lazing around in hotels or visits to hospitals or sit-ins at GP surgeries. If I could beg the odd bag of ice en route then so be it, but I wouldn't be going out of my way to find it. Finally I reminded everyone that somewhere in the UK today a grieving mother or father would have to explain to their kids that 'Daddy' or 'Mummy' had taken their own life and would never be coming home. I hoped this all too often occurring scenario in the veteran's community reiterated the seriousness of my cause. It certainly helped *me* to put my 'fun run' into perspective.

An enormous bridge appeared spanning a mile of seawater. Had I been up on my geography I'd have realised I was crossing the Dornoch Firth. If I'd gleaned up on my Scottish I'd have known that 'firth' means 'estuary'. As it was I crossed the imposing structure oblivious to both language and location yet filled with happiness and awe. It wasn't the longest bridge I'd ever traversed – that would be the one down in the Florida Keys – but it was the furthest crossing I'd made on foot. What an incredible adventure I was having.

Through the growing drizzle a sign for the Glenmorangie whiskey company appeared. You often put names to faces, but this was more a case of putting a place to a name. Connoisseurs of Scotch would hate me though, for although Glenmorangie's highland nectar is respected the world over, during my heavy drinking years I much preferred the cheap supermarket brands.

Despite the overcast umbrella and my ever-wetter kit and immense knee pain the running itself continued to present no problem. I trotted along without a care in the world, prepared to continue on through the gloom and well into the night. Only, a sign for LIDL made me rethink. I'd reached the outskirts of a village named Tein, having run an ultramarathon distance but still intent on clocking up another twenty miles. If I pitched camp now though the supermarket would be the ideal place to grab some breakfast and whatever else I needed.

I left the main road and set off across farmland, taking care to tread down the long grass to keep my trainers as dry as possible. I clambered over several barbed-wire fences until I found a suitable spot. To my surprise it overlooked the whiskey distillery itself and hundreds of oak barrels laid out in rows to the rear of the factory. A stunning rainbow spanning the ocean made up for the miserable weather – as did a steaming pot of broccoli soup and noodles and Ant's gripping audio book. A phone call from my former marine brother Gaz who'd recently emigrated to New Zealand was an additional bonus.

People's support was overwhelming, humbling and flattering, but it also got me thinking about the state of society and the future for my son. Why did everyone think this was such an amazing feat of endurance when to me, a mediocre runner with a busted back and zero training, it was obviously achievable? I guess the challenges I'd faced over the years had gifted me the ability to throw my mind, body and soul into the Batmobile whenever the call arose.

But there was more to it than that. When did risk adversity become so popular, not only in the workplace but in personal choice? Humans have been steered from our natural greatness in almost every way imaginable. Rather than rolling the sleeves up, getting stuck in and having a go, a worryingly high number of people in our fragmented and spiritually defunct communities now spend the majority of their precious spare time sitting on a comfortable sofa, gorging on mindless TV and proudly spouting off about things they 'won't do', 'couldn't do' and 'don't like' – when the underlying reality is our self-confidence and potential has been sapped by an evil corporate elite who manipulate our minds with their mainstream media, divide-and-control agenda and Hollywood scaremongering.

A poison such as alcohol is celebrated in Britain and yet eating a majority plant-based diet, one that rewards you with a focused mind, a wicked body, sound sleep and a happy life, is scoffed at – and usually by non-thinking naysaying Nigels who lack the open mindedness to try it. Mental health conditions are now viewed as badges of honour as opposed to the side effects of a toxic working environment, unhealthy human relations and living out of our egos instead of our hearts. Social media groups profess to offer support for these suffering souls and yet in reality indulge their misguided negativity as opposed to promoting a holistic approach to recovery comprising of properly proportioned nutrition, moderate exercise, meditation and positive self-talk.

My thoughts were only observations of present-day society and not a criticism of the individual. If folks are truly content in their everyday lives then I'm genuinely made up for them, but a quick surf of the Internet would suggest that this is often not the case. A statistically large number of people seem to float between simply existing and feeling anxious, guilty, depressed, inadequate and unfulfilled, all aspiring to an elusive utopian state but with no knowledge of how to go about achieving it.

Even on days when it's tempting to feel down I'm still overflowing with gratitude for my one chance on this beautiful blue planet. I will *always* insist on thinking of myself as the luckiest person on Earth. Why not? Positivity is free and plays a key role in your future wellbeing and that of those around you.

Monstering

Running is hard, but not running is harder.

Kermit T. Frog

Day 6 | Glenmorangie to Knockbain | 27.34 Miles

I woke up to a sunrise as spectacular as last night's sunset ... and a *sopping* wet tent – so waterlogged I had to wipe it down with my flannel-sized square of lightweight camping towel. During a Facebook video update, I sent the first page of the AA road map to Valhalla, setting it alight with a Clipper cigarette lighter worn on a loop of paracord around my neck.

After a LIDL breakfast consisting of a banana, cucumber, beef tomato and a packet of supergreens powder dissolved in a litre carton of coconut water, I tweeted a photo to Ant Middleton of me running along listening to his audio book. Ant retweeted my post with 'Good effort, buddy! One step at a time.'

Five miles down the A9 towards Inverness I slowed to a halt and plonked myself down on the verge at a T-junction. The agony from my knee was now too much to ignore and I needed anti-inflammatories to continue. Before doing so I wanted to find out what was wrong and for the umpteenth time began squeezing and probing my knee – but *nothing*.

I raked a fingernail over the kneecap – *'Ouch!'*

Pain rocketed around the joint.

Through a process of pinching and scratching I found that

a nerve beneath the skin was the insignificant source of so much discomfort. I surfed the Internet until I came across a lad posting about the exact same aggravation on a runners' forum. It came as a huge relief to realise the damage wasn't as serious as it felt. I popped a couple of 200mg ibuprofens, finished a conversation with a couple of friendly women out walking their dogs and saddled up.

A sign read 'Inverness 33' and I smiled, thirty-three in esoteric circles representing amongst other things enlightenment. I ran along checking my Facebook messages. One former marine had written, 'Royal, you better finish this fucking quickly. I've got cancer and a month to live'. I gave my brother my word I'd arrive at Land's End before he died and forwarded him some YouTube links for water-fasting and alkaline-living videos.

Another former commando Rob 'Brommers' Bromley, a mate from Nottingham, phoned to inquire how I was.

'Firing, brother!' I replied, relieved about my injury.

Brommers offered to coordinate the folks on Facebook who wanted to come and join me for a mile or two or provide food and accommodation. Many of them were former or serving bootnecks.

'Anyone is welcome to run with me, Rob, but ...'

This well-intentioned support could work in my favour, should I need a shower or to dry my equipment, but it might also seriously detract from achieving my goal. I told Brommers I didn't need a tidal wave of Lucozade or a barrage of burgers – a bowl of salad would be far more preferable – nor missionaries scouring the highways in an attempt to 'rescue' my poor exhausted soul.

I wasn't being ungrateful. I just didn't want to get roped into other people's agendas and have my mileage interrupted or dead animals and sugary shit shoved into my face.

As I entered a spotlessly clean roadside tearoom everyone inside turned and stared. I hadn't wanted to stop but my phone needed a charge and so I bought a baked potato and coleslaw and drank a lime and soda while waiting. The amiable female proprietor came over to ask what I was doing. I told her about my injured knee and plan to take eight 200mg ibuprofen a day, 'You can safely take four-hundreds,' she informed me.

The double dose made a huge difference, virtually no pain. Running past an off-duty oil rig sheltering in the estuary I grinned at the shear incredibleness and beauty of it all. A movement some distance away in a field caught my eye. An enormous feline-looking creature sprinted low over the wheat stubble before disappearing into a hedge. I managed to fire off a photo – the authentic big cat blurry type – and continued onwards wondering it if really was a panther or simply an effeminate dog.

I was running much faster, about a nine-minute-mile pace, not bad for a mid-life-crisis carrying half of Blacks Outdoors on his back. The grass on the verge was fairly short but still awkward and tiring to navigate. Instead I ran in the road, where I didn't have to pick my feet up as much. I threw appreciative nods and waves at the oncoming drivers, knowing the idiot quota would attempt to scare me onto the verge if I didn't. 'Flat Earth' someone had sprayed on back of a long road sign and I thought about my travels around this amazing planet and smiled.

As I began to cross another enormous span, the Cromarty Bridge, a van driver gave several friendly beeps of his horn. It was rewarding to realise people were getting to hear of my efforts. Now I was happily underway I hoped to find time to tweet to the media and get wider coverage for the fundraiser, which now stood at £2,000.

Darkness wasn't far off and so I stopped to brew a cuppa and eat a Caulder's Scottish Macaroon. Other than the coconut component I didn't know a great deal about macaroons, but this one looked and tasted like a tropical flapjack and it was delicious. I posed for a photo with Wolfie – a cuddly toy Harry had given me for company – knowing that in today's post-a-photo-of-your-pet climate the bean-filled canine would prove far more popular than me.

Two miles up a steep hill I answered my phone to Jenny. She wanted to know if it was a convenient time to tell Haz a bedtime story. It was an honour I never missed and so I ran the next two miles whilst narrating another epic Flying Thralls circus adventure. Running *and* storytelling – perhaps I could multitask after all.

Before leaving for Scotland I'd watched a YouTube video uploaded by a lad who'd trekked the length of the country. In the film he'd made a point of mentioning how increasingly *angry* he got with his surroundings as the trip progressed – the traffic, the trees, the bridges and the varying road surfaces. I had wondered if this Hulk-like phenomenon would affect me – and now it began to creep in. Not surprisingly it was the cars. Moreover the road-ragers inside them. Despite me having a fluorescent backpack cover and sporting a reflective flash on my running smock *and* two red-strobing lights, the majority of drivers still opted to *skim* past me even when the opposite carriageway was empty. I wasn't sure if I was angry at these dimwits or the state of humanity.

About eight miles from Inverness I'd entered ultra-distance territory and not wishing to risk further spinal damage in these early days, set about looking for a camping spot. An access road led up through a patch of woodland before cutting across sheep fields. I hopped the barbed wire fence behind the waist-high hedgerow and spent ten minutes selecting a spot out of sight of a distant light I assumed to be the farmhouse. I laid my headtorch in the grass so a limited beam lit an area the size of my tent's ground sheet and got the canvas up. I'd got in the habit of leaving the sole tent pole, it's five segments concertinaed, in the flysheet and the inner chamber clipped inside to save time.

One of the dog walkers from earlier Facebooked me to say well done and she'd donated to the cause, a much-appreciated gesture that brought a smile to my face. Then Taff Hillier from Radio Walkham in Devon messaged to invite me on his morning show sometime soon. Just as I brought my noodles to a boil the sound of a diesel engine grew louder and headlights lit up the tent.

Grabbing a corner of my sleeping bag I smothered the miniature LED light I used at night, turned off the gas and then sat there heart pounding as the vehicle drew near.

It stopped *right* by the tent.

Please ... please ... please ...

My anxiety shot through the roof up as I envisaged having to up-sticks and relocate my now-cosy self.

Fuck ... off!

I began to picture the 'scene' in *Deliverance,* Farmer Tavish McTavish and his toothless stable boy attempting to make me squeal like a pig – Yours Truly pointing out it's only a *1-man* tent in the hope they'd see sense and respect my personal space.

The vehicle drove off

Phew!

Through a gap in the zipped door I could just make out a

'Landrover' badge in the glow of the licence plate light. Ten minutes later the scenario *repeated* itself as yet another vehicle made its way back to the Old Chaparral.

Day 7 | Knockbain to Lewiston | 27.4 Miles

I woke up to a cup of tea but no food. I wasn't bothered – calories are overrated and runners tend to wet their pants over them. You can guarantee our hunter-gatherer ancestors went for days if not weeks without eating and still manged to cover colossal distances.

Five miles down the road the forest broke and the enormous Kessock Bridge into Inverness appeared in the distance. I happened across an American-style diner doing a roaring trade in not-so-American paninis. With no plant-based option on the cards, I opted for a couple of brie-filled offerings and a salad roll. Wolfing my choices down made me realise just how many calories I was burning. The food tasted so good and I ate double my usual amount.

In the breast pocket of my running smock the phone vibrated. Baz Gray had texted to ask where I was. I replied with 'Approaching Loch Ness', stowed the phone and didn't think any more of it.

The phone buzzed again. It was Sandy Nelson, another member of our Royal Marines brotherhood. We'd passed out of training together as 558 Troop originals. Sandy lived in Kilmarnock but business had brought him further north and he wanted to meet up to show his support. I fired off my location and began keeping half an eye out for the towering Scotsman.

I set off running again, shirtless in heaven-sent sunshine. I crossed the majestic bridge and for the first time on the trip navigation became an issue – due to a southerly phenomenon known as roundabouts. I hadn't needed the map so far – the A9 is the A9 is the A9 – and to be honest, what with having to faff about taking my rucksack off, I didn't want to now. I could have used the navigation app on my phone but was conscious of running the battery down. Instead I resorted to running around the outside of the roundabouts until I found the sign for Fort William.

My knee had twinged on the bridge and so it came as some relief to meet a cycling Aussie tourist, Ben, in Inverness, who told me I could safely ignore any strain-related pain.

At the northern end of Loch Ness hunger led me into in a quaint little establishment the Oakwood restaurant. By now I'd fathomed Scotland doesn't do vegetables – at least I hadn't found that menu option yet on my journey – and so went for the spaghetti bolognaise.

As I sat sipping tea from a bone-china service and popping ibuprofen the phone beeped. Baz again, wondering where I was now. I felt honoured the RSM was so concerned about my progress but surely my *exact* location wasn't important. I scrolled to Google Maps nonetheless, figuring Baz might be making a Facebook update on the Royal Marines page we co-hosted. Perhaps he was suggesting guys come and support me and needed an exact grid reference.

'Dochgarroch, mate' I replied, thinking no more of it.

Ten minutes later as I tucked into the tastiest spagbol ever cooked the bell above the restaurant door rang. I turned to see none other than the man *himself* approaching my table.

Jeeze! What are you doing here?' I chuckled.

How could it be my mate from Plymouth was *not only* up in Scotland but we'd opted for the *same* bloody eatery?

Then I remembered the text messages and it all fell into

place.

'Thought I'd see how you are.'

'Awh, thanks a million.'

Once a Royal Marine, always a Royal Marine – as our motto goes.

Baz hung my tent on his van to dry and took a photo of me in front of a giant hoarding with the words 'Loch Ness' emblazoned across it. I posted it to the #999miles Facebook page with the caption 'Today I get to swim with a legend – Nessie's words not mine', which garnered quite a response.

Baz laced up his runners and accompanied me south along the historic Loch. We ran in single file to avoid getting knocked down by the endless precession of campervans negotiating the narrow road's numerous blind bends. Every so often Baz would sprint ahead to film my progress for social media.

After ten miles Baz ran back to his own campervan. An hour and a half later he shot past me on his way to seek out a place to stop for the night. By the time I arrived in the shoreside village of Drumnadrochit the RSM had already pitched my tent in the rather ingeniously named 'Loch Ness Bay Camping' – the 'Bay' part so nobody could accuse the proprietor of lacking imagination.

I took my first shower in a week, one of those blissfully extended ones you enjoy when a business foots the bill. Then I joined my brother to post a live interview to the 999 Miles - Running from John O'Groats to Land's End Solo & Unsupported Facebook page. 'Chris has been reasonably fortunate with the weather so far,' said Baz, 'but the real challenge will start when he has nonstop rain for ten days and all his kit is soaking wet.'

I pondered these words, knowing that coming from an elite

soldier, a high-ranking mountain-and-arctic-warfare specialist, they were more likely a prediction than a possibility.

Baz kindly offered to buy supper. My stomach did the thinking for me and opted for a large fish and chips. 'Fancy a beer, mate?' he added.

'Nah, mate, I'm okay.'

Once again alcohol seemed so alien to me. I didn't miss it consuming my thoughts morning, noon and night, nor days lost to hangovers or the alcohol buzz itself.

Day 8 | Lewiston to Laggan | 32.14 Miles

And low and behold I found I didn't miss fish and chips either. The excess of rich protein and stodgy crabs sat heavily on my stomach all night and I woke up feeling as tired as when I went to sleep. A majority vegetable meal would have been digested in a third of the time, allowing my mind and body complete rest, the alkalinity enabling my tissues to detox and the vitamins revitalising my cells. As it was I felt lethargic, like I'd lost my mojo, and wished I could have been stronger-minded.

During the night my back had caused me significantly more pain than usual. With a month of ultramarathons in front of me this was a cause for concern. My worst fear was coming true but there was nothing I could do about it. Instead I put the anxious thoughts in an imaginary lead box and chucked it in the loch. While Baz the legend heated up beans and mash I did the interview over the phone with Taff at Radio Walkham.

Baz had brought along a Baton cap, T-shirt and promotional flag. Shunning tradition I'd decided not to carry the organisation's 'symbolic' baton, one fashioned from the sawn-off handle of a stretcher used on the battlefield in

Afghanistan. It had seemed nonsensical to spend hundreds of pounds on ultra-lightweight kit only to up the odds against me arriving at Land's End by shoving half a kilogram of rubber and steel into my bergen. I posted a photo on social media of me capped and flagged, then handed the items back to the RSM and kept the T-shirt.

Baz is one of the most humble and generous people I know and I loved and valued his company and sentiment. However, I'd been running along in a private trance-like furrow for days and hadn't anticipated the extent to which human contact would affect my single-minded focus. This was something I'd have to get used to as I wanted as many people as possible to get involved in the event.

Baz filmed me for a Facebook live as I ran off along the loch. I spent the first twenty minutes of the day conditioning my mind to expect more support along the way. I wasn't being a prima donna or ungrateful. It's just this was my dream, my horizontal 'Everest'. I'd invested a lot of time, money, family and myself in the venture and there was no way I could accept failure. Imagine making a summit attempt on that infamous Himalayan peak – only for a helicopter full of well-wishers to rock up and start suggesting different routes, meddling with your nutrition and altering your timings and equipment.

I ran through the forest fringing the Guinness-black loch and past the iconic Urquhart Castle, which must have featured in every Nessie-related production ever made. At lunchtime I pulled off the road and headed down a steep rocky incline to the water's edge. Baz had given me two hardboiled eggs, but no sooner had I washed them down with a cup of tea then tiredness overcame me and I lay back on my running smock and attempted a snooze.

It was no good. The beating sun turning my black smock

into a solar panel. I arose thirty minutes later from something far from sleep, more like a hangover in an oven, and got back on the road.

Even listening to Ant's inspiring audio book I was finding the running significantly harder today. I had zero energy and my legs felt like bags of cement. There was only one thing for it – stop moaning and go balls out.

I upped the pace to nine-minute miles and told myself to stop being a pussy as suicidal veterans were relying on me to stay alive, visualising my default and motivational image of a mother (or father) having to sit her kids down and explain daddy isn't coming home anymore as he's up there with the angels. This wasn't exaggeration or melodrama. A former Royal Marine with a wife and three children had topped himself only that week – another statistic to add to the 5,000 US veterans who'd killed themselves this year and the seventy-one in the UK.

The sad irony is that working through – or being supported to work through – tough experiences and mental health challenges results in a higher state of consciousness and a productive and balanced future. Looking back I wouldn't have traded my hardships for anything. The resulting vision enabled me to achieve all my goals and see through the bullshit in life, unlocking the essential quality of empathy along the way. If I could support one veteran to hang on in there and come through the other side then my efforts would be worth it.

I powered through my sluggish mindset and dead legs to run nineteen miles nonstop. With a deal of self-pride I arrived in the picture-postcard setting of Fort Augustus, a village centred on an enormous set of canal locks at the southern tip of Loch Ness. After gazing at Victorian-era terraces, neatly mown grass and plethora of gift shops, I ducked into the Turkish-run Moorings Restaurant and ate a delicious vegetable moussaka.

As the light faded, rain began to fall and so along with my headtorch I put on the ultralight Haglöfs jacket for only the second time this trip. Although a breathable, expensive and reputable brand, the waterproof had a plasticky texture, making me sweat and soaking my T-shirt in minutes. Pitch black now, I squeezed into the hedge to avoid an oncoming car. The vehicle stopped and a Monarch-of-the-Glen-type chappie wound his window down to ask if I wanted a lift. The odd road hog aside, Scottish people continued to be incredibly friendly.

In the drizzling blackness and shrouded by dense forest I made a Facebook Live update. Speaking from the heart I told the world how scared I was running in the dark past all these huge menacing trees without my mummy, adding that perhaps this whole John O'Groats escapade was a stupid idea. Bizarrely I didn't get the sympathy I'd hoped for – least not from the military community. Some veterans even employed such terms as 'nobber' – whatever that means.

Because Brommers would be posting my video to all of the Royal Marines-related Facebook pages, I'd added I would be arriving at the Commando Memorial in Spean Bridge around 11am if anyone wanted to come and meet me. I was pleased to be able to tell people I'd experienced the toughest day of running so far and my state of mind was still solid – I just had to trust my body would hold out. The update proved to be the most popular yet.

After thirty-three miles I was soaked to the core and began looking for a place to camp. The well-cut grass surrounding the Laggan swing bridge on Loch Oich looked perfect but was so close to the A82 that traffic noise and headlights would have plagued my sleep all night. I explored a couple of off-road spots, ending up knee-deep in bog water, before stopping at the start of the Great Glen Way. Although I looked forward to a bit of cross-country, this popular cycle track would add three miles to my trip. Cold, wet and tired I didn't want to commit to such a decision and decided to sleep on it. The only place to put the tent was on the cycle path's compacted grit surface. I pitched it off to the side in case any late-night bikers came through, hammering the pegs into the ground using a rock.

As I got the noodles and chopped veg on my phone rang. It was a former marine, a tough old sweat named Stuart Lavery, chairman of the 45 Commando Veterans Association. 'Chris, what are ye doon on the A82?' he bellowed in Jockwegian. 'It's *bloody* lethal! I'll pick you up in the morning and drop you somewhere safer.'

'I'm *fine,* mate.' I chuckled. 'I'm *running* not driving!'

'Need any dry socks?'

'I should be good,' I fibbed to save Stu any hassle – everything was wet bar my emergency kit.

I had a dream in which something didn't feel right ...

I was floating down a river in a cold wet cocoon ...

When the ringing in my head woke me at 4am I found to my horror I was!

The non-stop rain had loosened the surface of the cycle path and the tent pegs had pulled out. The majority of my kit had gone from damp to drenched – not only uncomfortable but potentially life threatening as I was due to enter the mountains today.

As with every other item of equipment my head torch had

a designated place in the tent. This way I knew where everything was and could save time packing my bergen each morning. I fumbled in a small draw-stringed kit bag for it, shoved my trainers on and then braved the maelstrom to secure my accommodation before it floated me to Land's End.

Over the Top

True leaders run at the back.

Skippy the Bush Kangaroo

Day 9 | Laggan to Fort William | 26.99 Miles

The wet and cold slowed my thinking and movement and I was slow to get going – or 'pull pole' to use marines' jargon. I had to leg it nonstop thirteen miles to Spean Bridge as I was already behind time for my 11am welcome party. Fortunately all those expectant faces put a spring in my step and I arrived only two hours late.

The memorial itself is impressive – a trio of granite-jawed commandos staring out over the rugged moorland while training to create havoc behind Hitler's lines. I pressed the Facebook Live button a quarter-mile from the statue and gave a speech about the commandos' legendary values, how these men knew they likely wouldn't return from their dagger-in-the-teeth missions and yet volunteered anyway, how the commando ethos helped me to hold my own while battling the horrors of chronic drug addiction.

I weaved around the milling tourists and paused my broadcast to salute the men of stone high up on the plinth. Then I turned to greet my welcome committee of ... *no one!*

I wasn't bothered or surprised. I'd only announced my ETA late last night and hadn't expected anyone to drop what they were doing to drive all the way out here. I was simply happy to have arrived, though somewhat disconcerted about the constant downpour. It was time to go and find the breakfast I should probably have eaten before running a half marathon whilst starving, piss-wet through and carrying the weight of a widescreen television.

I made my way towards the village and came across the Spean Hotel. From one side of the premises a huge serving hatch produced boxes of fish and chips for groups of walkers congregated at open-air picnic tables. *'Brrrhh!'* I shivered and made my way inside, delighted to find an inhouse commando museum.

After perusing the nostalgia on display I took a seat in what was more a functional eating hall than a ye-olde highland restaurant. Unable to find a vegetable option on the menu, I ordered chicken and chips with mushy peas and curry sauce plus *two* deserts. In my sodden condition the food went down a treat, the Romanian waiter laughing to find me drying my socks on my shoulders beneath my running smock. He said I was welcome to hang my sleeping bag and tent out across a couple of chairs.

It was a miserably wet nine miles to Fort William and I ran all the way to fend off hypothermia. Thoughts of the West Highland Way occupied my mind, a route I felt fairly certain I would take. One of the guys I'd met at John O'Groats had walked 'The Way' and from what he'd said, along with information on the Internet, I envisaged an idyllic moorland trail dotted with pubs and hostels. 'Oh, I walked it last year,' said Per, a Swede working in the petrol station I stopped at. 'You should be okay.'

Sorted, I thought, stocking up on powdered milk, a pot noodle and snacks.

Arriving in the bustling tourist town of Fort William,

nestled in the folds of Ben Nevis, I was slightly disconcerted by a white-hand-painted bike padlocked to a fence, courtesy of www.ghostbikes.org, a rather haunting tribute to Jason MacIntyre, killed at this junction in 2008. Apparently these junked bikes act as both a memorial and a reminder to motorists to look out for cyclists.

'The original end of the West Highland Way' a sign greeted me. 'Congratulations from the Ben Nevis Highland Centre – now come inside and buy your certificate.'

I smiled. How narrowminded to assume pilgrims only travelled north – and as for *buying* your own certificate, I thought only phony TEFL teachers did that on the Khao San Road!

Now I was faced with yet another decision as it was getting dark and *still* raining but I had mileage left in my legs. Should I find a cheap hostel here in Fort William in which to dry all my gear or would I be better off taking a gamble and heading straight down the Yellow Brick Road? My ultralight fleece, woolly hat and tracksters were still safely waterproofed in my bergen in case of emergency, my sleeping bag now only a third sodden, but reports were saying it was close to freezing up on the high ground tonight. I had to avoid becoming so wet and cold I couldn't get the tent up before being overcome by hypothermia. The same went for keeping my reserve clothing and down sleeping bag dry, which in that one-man water trap was easier said than done. In view of my ridiculously low body fat as a result of the water fast either scenario could mean certain death.

I continued onwards but reminded myself of the unspoken promise I'd made to my boy not to put our relationship in jeopardy. I had a compass to prevent me getting disorientated should heavy fog come down and so long as I made certain I was definitely on the trail I could leg it at least thirty miles in one hop to civilization if necessary.

My concerns were well-founded, for the poorly marked track proved impossible to locate initially. Luckily for me a Japanese woman in a poncho, rucksack and walking boots came stomping out of the forest fifty metres away– *Ahhh!* It must have taken her all day to walk from Kinlochleven, the nearest village along the route, confirming that at this late hour I'd have to spend a night under canvas.

After six miles of running up the slopes of Ben Nevis I came across a thistle symbol on a small wooden post. Obviously the thistle represented *a* trail but was it *the* trail? There was no Internet signal on my phone and so I had no way of finding out. My confusion stemmed from the path being no different to a muddy sheep track, whereas the rocky one I'd followed so far was as wide as a main road. Both appeared to head in the right direction but it was hard to tell on the rudimentary AA map which was the West Highland Way.

The rainfall morphed into buckets, forcing me to focus on getting the tent up sharpish. But it took an age to find a level spot, one without sharp stones or thistles that could penetrate the tent's groundsheet and puncture my lightweight Thermarest mattress. I was conscious of only having four 'lives' in the form of sticky patches to repair it.

Day 10 | Fort William to Devil's Staircase | 20.44 Miles

Fortunately the sky stayed open all night so Mother Nature could empty all of the water out of it. Closing the zip on the flysheet two thirds trapped most of the moisture from my mystery-illness sweats and breath, which then dripped onto the sleeping bag, worsening my predicament. I leant on one arm in the cramped tent, sipping tea and peering at the sheeting rain, recalling the RSM's words: 'But the real challenge will start when Chris has nonstop rain for ten days.' Being September I'd anticipated a little drizzle and the occasional short-lived downpour, but I genuinely hadn't expected such a constant deluge. The blissful days of sunshine in the North now seemed so far removed.

I couldn't stay in the tent again tonight with a wet sleeping bag without risking hypothermia. My options included going back to Fort William to dry off – I'd rather not – or running the ten miles or more to Kinlochleven nonstop over mountainous terrain. I say nonstop because that would ensure my core temperature didn't drop to a dangerous level. I had no margin for error though. If I took a wrong turn and got lost or injured I had no dry camping gear in which to take refuge.

The heavy shower eased and after drying my socks in the cooking pan and using the last wet wipe I decided to go for it. I packed up my equipment and settled into a steady jog, concentrating on not turning an ankle on the rock-strewn terrain. After three miles the trail entered a large logging area ... and then finished.

Damn!

I'd reached the end of a steep-sided gulley and there was no path out of it. The bloody thistle sign *had* been a marker for the West Highland Way. I couldn't risk backtracking and adding six useless miles to the day's tally, not when getting my shivering tired state to Kinlochleven was a matter of urgency. There was only one thing for it – I'd have to climb a hundred-and-fifty-metres up the forty-five-degree incline to get back on course. It would be no easy task because hundreds of felled tree trunks littered the slope, like a monster-sized version of the pick-up-sticks game. Carrying a heavy pack I was acting in my very own Rambo movie – the one where John-J gets piss-wet cold in a shit tent in Scotland and wishes he had a helicopter and a hot bath. My heart pumped anxiety around my body. I felt dangerously out on a limb and couldn't wait to have the West Highland Way safety beneath my Karrimors.

I made the slippery climb without mishap, yet wasted a lot of unnecessary energy in the process. It came as quite some relief to see four hikers ambling along the 'correct' trail, all of them clad in Gore-Tex waterproofs and gaiters and with sturdy leather boots on their feet.

Not so reassuring was the large boggy pool between me and them. Having gone to great lengths not to let my waterproof training shoes get flooded I wasn't going to take my eye off the ball now. I began leaping from rock to gorse clump to rock, eventually landing on the West Highland Way with a supersized sense of relief.

A mile further on, the narrow gorse-hedged path left the forest and opened into a track the size of a country lane, one that snaked upwards into highlands. Shortly after an unexpected water obstacle appeared. There'd been so much rain – still was so much rain – a shin-deep stream now ran down from the mountains and across the trail.

Shit!

I recalled a trek my team completed on an expedition to Iceland. We'd all had Teva sandals strapped to our backpacks for just this eventuality.

Having dismissed the idea of wading across barefoot I hopped onto a boulder half an inch below the surface. As I picked out my next stepping stone a Swedish couple approached from the opposite direction. 'Oh ...' Sven shook his head. 'There's another fifty of these rivers between here and Kinlochleven.'

'Tack så mycket,' I thanked him and smiled.

Then with a shrug I stepped into the mini-torrent and waded purposely across as more hardcore hikers passed me on their way south, all determined strides, hardy smiles and rain-proofing as they tore up the hills.

A few things struck me. The first being that in the two conversations I'd had with people about the possibility of taking the West Highland Way no one had considered I was wearing flimsy running shoes – including myself. I didn't belong here, for in my super-tired state negotiating the rocky ground was hard work. Nor did I like being so exposed in bad weather with such inappropriate kit knowing one wrong turn could be my downfall. At least on the road it was nigh-on impossible to get lost and I had the option of flagging down a vehicle in an emergency.

Kinlochleven is home to the world's largest ice-climbing wall and was the first village in the world to connect every house to electricity. I made up my mind to book into a backpacking hostel when I arrived and make full use of the drying room and facilities. It would mean only completing ten miles today, so I'd have to make up the lost ultramarathon distance somewhere down the line.

Three hours later as I trotted down a forest trail into the lakeside settlement, I saw a sign declaring 'Black Water Hostel. 500 Metres' nailed to a tree. Outside the hostel I noted rows of soaking wet tents on a patch of flooded grass. A shiver ran down my spine. I certainly wouldn't be taking Black Water's budget option.

A sign on the reception desk read 'Closed between 1-2pm'. I checked my Casio – 13:02hrs.

Acht!

I had an idea …

Taking a mosey around the back of the building I found a portacabin housing the drying room. I sprang into action as fast as my numb fingers allowed. Having squared away the jumble of already dried kit strewn across the racks, I hung up my wet camping equipment, switched on a large dehumidifier and turned the heaters to full. Within ten minutes the place was a stinky sauna but I wasn't complaining. Compared to the misery of the last forty-eight hours my newly warm state was sheer bliss. Besides, if I could get my gear dry I was safe to set out across the mountains this afternoon.

What a *result!* I packed my kit away, checked the map and decided to push over the highlands to meet the main A82 at Altnafeadh aka 'The Devil's Staircase'. The route was nine miles – seven shorter than taking the road via Glencoe. It would mean running 1,021 metres up Buachaille Etive Mor in a pair of shorts, a significant obstacle when you consider the peak of Ben Nevis is 1,345 metres. The sky was completely clagged over making it prematurely dark. I'd likely be the last person on the mountain trail and with no phone signal, giving me zero margin for error. However having a dry sleeping bag should I need to bivouac in an emergency gave me the confidence to set forth.

The trail out of Kinlochleven soared upwards like a rollercoaster through the low-lying forest. Bang on cue the sky opened and rain fell like swimming pools. I whipped off the running smock and, now topless, pulled the Haglöfs jacket from the bergen's flap pocket, where I kept it for rapid deployment. Within seconds the waterproof's clammy plastic-like material had me dripping in sweat. So long as I didn't stop running though I could keep hypothermia at bay in the approaching sub-zero temperature.

Leaving the treeline to enter knee-high heather I realised I faced several serious problems. The trail was now a fast-flowing ankle-deep stream and I had no choice but to slosh on through. Visibility worsened as moisture saturated the air. You only have to become disoriented in fog *once* in your life to understand how terrifying and deadly this can be. Making matters worse, should I run into difficulties there was nowhere to pitch the tent as the path was underwater and everything else either bog or springy heather. It was only because I had the compass and an impossible-to-miss road to my south that I decided to continue.

The whole situation just scraped below the idiotic part of ridiculous. I'm only half-stupid and had no intention of dying on this hill – but it felt bloody near to it. For the first time on the trip I felt massively sad for Jenny and Haz. They'd be at home now on a warmish evening in Plymouth sitting on the couch watching cartoons while the little man of the house ate his tea. Little did the two of them know the gamble I was taking with their future happiness.

Alone, bitterly cold in a pair of shorts, carrying a house on my back in a washing machine on one of Scotland's highest peaks, having to run or die, I can honestly say I wanted out of this off-road trekking malarkey. It came as a massive relief when three hours later I descended the monster-sized rocks making up the Devil's Staircase and the A82 came into view.

As predicted, when I stopped running the initial stage of hypothermia kicked in. I whacked on my dry smock, tracksters and woolly hat but it was no good. My core temperature had plummeted to the point where I needed a heat source to rewarm. I *had* to get the tent up and the cooker on fast. I headed to the only flat grassy spot for miles around, paying token attention to the small misted-up campervan parked on it.

Two lads who from the shorts and trail shoes they wore appeared to be distance runners – the Kinlochleven Ultramarathon took place earlier today – were busy putting up their own tent. The diamond guys broke from what they were doing to come and help me out – only unfamiliar with my tent's setup there wasn't much they could do. With cold-deadened fingers and brain fog I took a worrying age to get the canvas up, my teeth chattering like those wind-up ones sold in joke shops.

Fuck ...!

Noooo ...!

Unstrapping the sleeping bag from the base of my pack I could tell it was *drenched*. The stuff sack Baz had lent me to replace my Lidl carrier bag obviously wasn't waterproof. I could have *sworn* it was – there was no way I'd have carried my lifesaving sleeping bag outside the bergen if not.

Now I had a real dilemma. My five-hundred-quid tent was soaked inside and out and I didn't have the option of crawling into my three-hundred-quid sleeping bag to rewarm. I could always reach out to the two lads or in a worst-case scenario flag down a passing motorist, but I didn't want to unless absolutely necessary. I began fumbling with the cooker to get some heat into my waterlogged tomb.

'*Knock-knock!*' came a Scottish man's friendly voice. 'Fancy a cup of coffee?'

The United Nations, Bono and Father Ted gathered in Geneva to discuss this most outlandish of propositions ...

YES, HE FUCKING WELL DOES! was their diplomatic response.

'Awh, *mate,* that would be awesome!' I replied through the flimsy green fabric.

'Cool. We're in the van.'

Duncan and Jayne were the most decent and hospitable natives you could ever hope to meet. They smothered me in sweaters, blankets and dogs and poured fresh coffee and shoved cakes down my throat. Had it been my drinking days a dram of the Highland nectar would have hit several spots right about now. As it was I didn't even think about it.

The caring couple offered to drive me back to the Black Water Hostel, a practical and tactical withdrawal so to speak. In the epic scheme of running #999miles it was the sensible option and staying here to freeze certainly wasn't. I'd just have to hitchhike back to the Devil's Staircase in the morning.

Jenny the manager at Black Water continued the Scottish trend of bending over backwards to help me ... the only issue being they didn't have any rooms. Nor did any other place in town when she kindly phoned around on my behalf. 'It's gunnae have to be the camping.' She nodded at the rows of miserable tents floating around on the semi-submerged field. 'But I'll get you a dry sleeping bag.'

I was still shivering and the lure of a wet tent compared to a heated room with a fluffy duvet and stinking-hot shower was about as appealing as smallpox.

After fetching me the sleeping bag Jenny began to lock the office.

The phone rang.

'One sec.' She dived back inside.

Seconds later, 'You're in luck!' Jenny beamed. 'A group of clients just cancelled, so you've gottae four-person room to yourself.'

Day 11 | Devil's Staircase to Tyndrum | 24 Miles

Having woken up happy in a cloud of duvet and pillows, a

little dehydrated as I'd abused the novelty of having my very own heater in the spotless dorm, I opened the window to draw off the miasma emanating my running smock. Ordinarily I would have taken advantage of the hostel's facilities and handwashed the jacket before going to sleep, but by the time I'd showered and hung almost every item of kit up in the drying room it was approaching midnight.

There was a large group of smiling and bowing Japanese ultrarunners staying at the backpackers. After they'd slipped off to bed I obeyed the sign in the kitchen ordering me to 'Help yourself to any food in this cupboard'. Inside was a veritable Fortnum and Mason for trekkers and before long I was tucking into a large saucepan full of pasta in Dolmio sauce with abandoned vegetables.

At 0900hrs the hospitality Jenny the manager had shown me had the haggis kicked out of it by a grumpy old bastard who interrupted my breakfast of porridge and bananas to tell me to check out.

'I didn't get in until late,' I told him. 'Give us ten more minutes, will you?'

'The cleaners need to clean the room,' he continued.

They hadn't even arrived yet.

'So be *quick* as you can.'

So in a hostel with fifteen rooms they need to clean mine first, you fucking jobsworth!

I ignored him, throwing on my smock to go out and buy ibuprofen and a bin liner to waterproof the sleeping bag.

With my technical, medical, outdoor and wash kit organised in small piles around the room, I collected the tent, sleeping bag and clothing from the drying room. Then I set about packing in a logical fashion, binning any unused item, like blister tape and mosquito repellent, stuff I could buy en route if required. I had a Facebook message from my recruit buddy Sandy Nelson, the third now, asking where I'd be around 5pm. I replied with the A82 around Loch Tulla, wishing I could be more specific, only my mind was focused on reaching Land's End.

Fulton McKay popped his angry head around the door and began growling about birds falling from the sky and earthquakes in Dundee because I hadn't vacated my room. Then the chancer hopped into a four-by-four and drove off – so I went for a shower. When I finally left the backpackers at midday ... the cleaners still hadn't arrived.

In the ice-climbing centre's equipment shop I found a pair of breathable Gore-Tex bottoms. I hadn't been able to wear my tracksters to keep warm because the rain would have soaked them immediately and put me in even more danger. By carrying these Gore-Tex over-trousers and having my sleeping bag properly waterproofed I could prevent a repeat performance of yesterday's hypothermic fiasco. Figuring Jen and I had spent more than enough of our savings I decided to take Alan up on his offer to pay for my unforeseen expenses. Over the phone he kindly put the ice-climbing centre's somewhat extortionate fee of £125 on his credit card.

It was day four of the continued downpour. Clad in my waterproofs I stuck a thumb out and a seasoned fellow traveller Fiona picked me up in her 2CV and dropped me at the Devil's Staircase.

That's where the day's pleasantness ended. It was the heaviest rain I've experienced outside of monsoons in the Tropics, with winds gusting up to what must have been eighty miles an hour. Each time an articulated lorry passed by on the barren highland road I had to crouch down and grab the crash barrier to prevent the draw of the monster-sized rig sucking me under its wheels. Having lifted the floodwater off the tarmac the truck would then spew it out of its wake and all over me.

After five miles I was in dire need of a cuppa but no such establishment appeared bar a sole hotel too far off the A82 to make it worth the detour. I passed a strangely out-of-place construction site and wondered what sort of welcome I'd receive if I knocked on the builders' portacabin and asked to use the kettle – I'm sure it would have been a warm Scottish one.

The windchill penetrated my Haglöfs rain jacket and so I slipped my running smock on underneath – I'd binned my two T-shirts. The smock soon became saturated in sweat but the waterproof acted like a wetsuit, keeping me warm – so long as I kept moving. If forced to stop for any reason I'd have about ten minutes before the wetsuit effect morphed into a fridge-like one. This made for a massive trust exercise as I had to have the self-belief that I could run twenty-four miles nonstop to a place called Tyndrum – there didn't appear to be any other civilisation on the map.

I jogged along scanning my surroundings for a place to pitch the tent in an emergency. There was nothing – except waist-high heather as far as the eye could see. Worse still there were no farm buildings or even a single tree to shelter under should things get serious. I put my head down and ran through the storm, only stopping briefly to flick the Vs at a sign declaring 'End of the Highlands'.

Running past Loch Tulla I added an enormous dull-eyed deer to the mental inventory of roadkill I'd compiled, a list that now comprised of bats, falcons, slowworms, stoats, weasels, squirrels, hedgehogs, cats and more badgers than you can shake a stick at (although technically that's badger-baiting which is an imprisonable offence).

The random assortment of junk on Britain's roadsides was also an eye-opener. You can kit yourself out in a whole wardrobe of fluorescent yellow safety gear plus several choices of helmet. There's enough food wrappers and drinks containers to make the education system proud and so many license plates you could register every car on the M25. Oh, and if you're ever in need of a hole punch there's one sitting on the kerb just outside Invermoriston.

After eighteen miles I came upon an advertising sign for the Bridge of Orchy Hotel boasting 'Real ales, real fire, real food, real bridge'. I could do with some 'real' respite from the elements as well as the biggest plate of food ever served in the hamlet's 267-year history. The majestic white hotel turned out to be a popular trekker stop-off and had more waterproofs than Go Outdoors hanging on a coatrack in its mega-plush bar.

'Kitchen's closed,' said the barman. 'We've only got cake.' He nodded to one of those silver-tiered Victorian things loaded with brown spongey wedges that may well have been appetizing had I not craved something savoury.

'Nothing else?'

'Just cake.' He frowned.

'Well … *cake* it is then.' I smiled. '… and six packets of salt-and-vinegar, please.'

Tyndrum lay seven miles south, the barman saying there were several backpacking hostels and campsites there. It had gone 8pm and I was tired. I necked my … *cake* and began slogging onwards, passing Lord-of-the-Rings-like peaks ringed by pine forest. Through the perma-drizzle Tyndrum's legendary Green Welly diner finally came into view. Alan had mentioned this place when I called to thank him again for the waterproof bottoms. Wearing them over my shorts had not only kept my legs dry but ventilated and warm – a real result.

I followed signs for the 'By the Way Hostel' but somehow managed to run right out of town. I backtracked but was only able to find 'The Pines Trees Caravan and Camp Park'. *Maybe I've misunderstood something,* I thought, wandering into the grounds in the hope of finding a backpacker dormitory.

As I peeked into the camp site's shower block – attempting to sum up whether these particular showers were showery enough for my liking – a voice gruffed, *'Ruhh-ruh-rurhr-ruh?'*

I turned to see it was Grizzly Adams inquiring into my welfare. I'm not sure where his bear was – I think he might have eaten him.

'I was looking for the hostel,' I replied, wondering if the mountain man would be interested in trading a leg of moose for some water-purification tablets.

'Ruh-ruh-rurrh-ruh-rurrrh.'

He began walking towards a caravan.

Assuming this was the reception I tagged on behind, looking forward to a warm dry room or at least a cosy bunk.

Inside the caravan something seemed amiss. Football played on a big TV in what appeared to be a living area, a half-drunk pint of beer on the side. But it wasn't until Grizzly Adams turned around and promptly jumped a foot in the air – impressive for a big lad – that I realised this was his actual home.

Scowling like a scorned Viking he jabbed a finger out. *'Rurhh-rurh-ruh road!'*

Feeling only massively stupid, I figured I was in the wrong place – unless I needed to skin a beaver or smoke some possum jerky.

When I finally located the By the Way Hostel the

reception had closed, leaving me no choice but to sail my tent on their quagmire and beg someone for the bathroom code. *Still,* I consoled myself over a Pot Noodle and instant mash, *at least I won't have to pay the camping fee.*

Highlander

If you wanna be my lover, you better run with my friends.

Frank Bruno

Day 12 | Tyndrum to Firkin Point | 27.25 Miles

I woke up purposely early only to find my mattress had a slow puncture and was half inflated – or deflated, depending upon your outlook on life. It wasn't a major issue as I was always so exhausted that I woke up in the same position I fell asleep in. I could have patched the leak but getting on the road took priority. Before that though I made a moral charity-based decision to quietly ignore the 'Don't dry your tent or sleeping bag' sign in the drying room.

I couldn't brew a cuppa as the hostel's water was brown and the sterilisation tablets needed an hour to take effect. Instead I moved my operation over to the Green Welly and in the absence of anything remotely plant-like on the menu, opted for a bacon sandwich and the Scotland's worst Wi-Fi instead.

After running until midday and banking eighteen miles I arrived on the fabled shores of Loch Lomond, which I could have sworn was the birthplace of Connor MacLeod the 'Highlander'. As such it came as something of a disappointment to realise Loch Lomond's not even *in* the Highlands – it's in the Trossachs, which doesn't even sound Scottish.

I sat on a bench at the Inveruglas Visitor Centre, brewing a cup of tea and chatting to two delightful female German artists, Ully and Nena, as the Loch Lomond pleasure boat loaded up with fun-loving tourists. After half hour of loch-based banter during which we covered all aspects of deep black water surrounded by bushy trees, the girls invited me stay in their holiday cottage. Ully added, 'Scottish houses are *very* freezing!'

With more distance to do I gratefully declined and went to fill up my water bladder for the third time this day. To avoid carrying unnecessary weight I never put more than a litre in – except when approaching my camping spot. This time I was out of luck. A sign in the toilet read 'Not for Drinking!' Fortunately the staff in the café handed me two half-litre bottles free of charge the second I asked.

After twenty-three miles I was about two thirds of the way along the lake. I came across a derelict restaurant all boarded up bar one smashed window. I peered inside to find the place eerie but habitable and with only a light sprinkling of bat shit on the floor. In the end I decided to give it a miss as I had more mileage in my legs. Worryingly I didn't have such distance in my back, which was now extremely sore.

Approaching the first piece of pavement I'd seen on the trip outside of town centres, I shifted the weight of the bergen onto my hips. It did nothing to reduce the pain and so reluctantly I began keeping an eye out for a camp spot. Firkin Point, a pebbly strip of beach dotted with trees, would be ideal. Unable to drive in a tent peg, I wrapped the guy ropes around some of the bigger stones and piled smaller ones on top.

In a Facebook Live update I informed my growing bunch of loyal supporters that my little toes were infected and right knee double the size. I added that along with my sciatica at DEFCON 5 I was covered in prickly heat bumps and mosquito bites. I ended the video on a positive with, 'So the pain is telling me I'm not trying hard enough.'

Lying in the tent listening to the gently lapping waves I congratulated myself on visiting the birthplace of the Highlander – even if the film should really have been called the *Lowlander*. Little did I know Hollywood had actually got it right because the immortal sword-wielding Scotsman was actually born further north on the shores of Loch Shiel.

Day 13 | Firkin Point to Paisley | 27 Miles

Whoop-whoop!

Hands up who's got a dry tent – *Me!*

With no downpour last night I was able to leave the flap open and the breeze wafting across Loch Lomond's dark ruffled waters blew out all the moisture.

The yang to my perma-happy ying was some of the responses to last night's Facebook update, comments such as 'You've raised awareness of veteran suicide so you can go home now' and 'Why don't you book into a hotel for a few days – you've got nothing left to prove'.

I understood the majority of these people meant well but their ill-thought-out and off-the-cuff replies were devaluing the ultramarathon a day challenge I'd set myself, along with the investment, effort and fortitude. One woman even *ordered* me to give her my location so she could travel seven hundred miles to take over the running!

I'd already told my supporters that these 'pain' reports were solely to keep them in the loop and not me seeking attention or an excuse to give up. I thought the Facebook followers and media companies would be interested to hear how my body was holding up as the mileage accumulated. You never see an endurance-sport documentary where the doubt-ridden contender doesn't have to overcome at least one mental or physical hurdle – usually whilst blubbering over how much they miss their family.

My intention had been to give people a sense of the adversity I faced and hopefully raise more money for the charity. But if the usual offenders continued to try and persuade me to stop I'd clam up about my niggles and arrive at Land's End regardless.

I received yet another message from Sandy and felt bad I couldn't be more specific with respect to a rendezvous. Upon hitting the road I was pleased my back pain held off ... for the first five miles.

While indulging in a 'Full Monty' breakfast at the plush Inn on Loch Lomond, I made a Facebook update about the heels on my two-week-old Karrimor trail shoes – or the lack of them. The specialist I'd seen about my peroneal tendonitis reckoned I had unusually high arches, which meant although I landed on my forefeet, like a true Kenyan champ, the outsides of my heels scraped the ground first, wearing my shoes out prematurely and costing me a fortune.

No sooner had I posted a photo of the trainers to social media then offers to buy me a new pair came flooding in – only as absurd as it may sound I didn't have the time or focus to enter into such a dialogue. Instead I called my buddy George in Glasgow and asked him to grab me some more Karrimors from Sports Direct. I'd arranged to stay with George tonight and so this kept things simple.

The next stretch of the A82 towards Clydebank proved to be insanity perfected, a full-on-and-hectic dual carriageway with a verge too overgrown to run on. According to Google Navigator there was no alternative route, leaving me no option but to set off facing the oncoming traffic. Every time an articulated lorry approached I stepped off the road, the drivers of these enormous rigs waving to thank me for acknowledging their limited manoeuvrability. I passed a sign for a place called 'Renton' and smiled. Then the outskirts of Dumbarton loomed and needing water and a bite to eat I entered a service station –

And literally *bumped* into Sandy!

It was great to see my recruit training brother and kind of him to treat me to a Subway meal and make a generous donation to the Baton. Shame it was such a short meeting but on the bright side our troop had regular reunions.

In this urban environment I began using the walking route function on Google Navigator. Surprisingly accurate, it led me along a cycle path next to the Forth and Clyde Canal in the direction of Clydebank. Passing brightly painted cruisers moored in an idyllic granite basin surrounded by neatly mown grass, enormous bushy trees and architecture and ironwork that would have made Fred Dibnah proud, I was on Cloud Nine. The running came easy and as my eyes smiled at the ducks and swans paddling amongst the reeds my mind looked forward to seeing an old friend.

George and I met in 2003 on an access-to-university course when we discovered a shared passion for surfing. With the exception of my media appearances he's the only person who has ever asked me what happened in Hong Kong. For six years I'd shrugged off losing a million-dollar business and taken the trauma of addiction, the triads and psychosis on the chin, but George was so interested and such a good listener that we delayed diving into the waves for four hours while I told him everything. People often ask me if writing *Eating Smoke* was therapeutic. I say no – digging up stuff that should remain in the past has had exactly the opposite effect – but talking to George was definitely an experience I'd describe as healing.

With this morning's social media responses still gnawing away at my all-important positivity, I decided to silence the bad vibes once and for all with some reverse psychology. At the end of the afternoon's Facebook Live broadcast I *promised* everyone I would run an ultramarathon a day to Land's End, that I *would* see my boy at the finish line and nothing could possibly stop me. I added that pain was always going to be a part of a challenge like this and suggested if folks truly wanted to support me they should do so with encouragement rather than dissuasion – thus making everyone shareholders in my success.

It garnered exactly the response I intended, replies such as '99.9% could not do this. You can. It's simple, Royal' and 'It's a challenge – of course it fucking hurts!' and 'Crack on, Chris. Land's End. Nonstop. End of!' all of which made me smile. But perhaps the biggest boost of all, 'What a lucky boy your son is.'

Day 14 | Paisley to Wishaw | 28 Miles

George, his partner Leigh and their two young girls lived in a village just outside Paisley. A Radox bath did wonders for my mind, only the hot water made my legs swell considerably. I wasn't complaining though. George and Leigh looked after this weary pilgrim extremely well *and* fed me a huge and delicious salad.

Despite my nightly soaking, I genuinely didn't mind staying in the tent but looked forward to a solid sleep on the guys' sofa bed nonetheless. Unfortunately it wasn't to be because my fever kicked up, drenching me in sweat and unusually I had a horrendous nightmare.

In the morning I headed for Achilles Heel, a popular running shop on the edge of Glasgow City Centre. My feet had swollen so much I couldn't get them into the Karrimors George had bought me. Plan B, I'd take the manager of Achilles Heel up on her offer of support, kindly coordinated by a Facebook supporter.

By the time I'd covered the seven miles into the city I had shooting pains up the back of my calves as a result of the worn-out trainers. Had Achilles Heel been any further I would have binned the shoes and gone barefoot. As it was I donated them to the shop's charity collection and ran off in an especially comfortable pair of Brooks – the only issue being they weren't waterproof.

Today I would be straying slightly east to hook up with another good mate, Scottish Dave, a guy I'd trained to work in Sub-Saharan Africa with. Dave lived in Wishaw, a little over marathon distance away according to the navigator.

Perfect.

I set off through the centre of Glasgow.

A Co-op sign loomed and I suddenly felt hungry.

I hopped inside the shop, figuring a falafel wrap or sandwich-type device would stoke the fire for a while.

A grey-haired chap in a dark suit and tie beamed at me like a vicar.

Rather well dressed for the Co-op ...?

Something didn't seem right.

I took a look around the *mauve-and-grey* establishment, spotting a sign offering 'Fitting tributes in the event of a loss' and a smartly framed poster comparing prices with rival body snatchers such as 'Dignity'.

Realising I wasn't in Kansas anymore I backed out of the door and crossed the road to a pizza place, where I bought a soggy slice of mozzarella that really *did* need cremating.

It wasn't only an ibuprofen tablet welded to the back of my throat giving me problems today. The voice on my phone, 'Sat Nav Woman' as I thought of her, kept telling me to take the first exit at roundabouts when the correct route was straight on. Luckily for me a quick check of the electronic map confirmed the right way.

As I ran through Glasgow's historic centre Stuart Lavery called to see how I was. It sounded as if he was in the car with a load of barrel-chested bald men. 'Do you wannae lift south? We're onae way to Lympstone for a troop reunion!' he joked.

'No thanks, Stu.' I chuckled.

I continued on towards Wishaw, noting how the unparalleled beauty of the lochs and highlands had melded into one vast nondescript urban sprawl interspersed with the odd bit of greenery – a tree, a privet hedge, a strip of grass or a playground. For all I knew I might have been passing through thriving hubs of industry, but these areas seemed more like post-eighties' government investment fudges intended to pacify communities experiencing rampant unemployment.

One of the wonderful things about Scotland is that when you pause to check directions passers-by stop and ask you if you're okay. When I explained my mission to one such chap in Bellshill, he informed me he was off to complete his *El Camino* pilgrimage in Spain the next day and insisted on paying for my lunch. I popped into the Belmill Hotel to be greeted by a lot of expensive-looking whiskies but none of the *haute cuisine* the place is famous for. Their kitchen had stopped serving and so I ordered two packs of salt-and-vinegar and a pint of lime and soda instead.

I arrived in Wishaw soaking wet and tank on empty. With twenty-six-and-a-half miles in the bag I was pleased to have nudged – albeit tokenistic – into ultramarathon territory and content to call it a day. But when I typed Scottish Dave's address into the phone, I found he lived a mile and a half out of town. I didn't mind. I seemed to be immune to running and pressed on listening to Sat Nav Woman's dulcet but misleading tones. In a Tesco Express at the end of Dave's road I bought an enormous Quorn lasagne, stuffed it into my bergen and located his house.

Scottish Dave was a long-distance lorry driver and wouldn't be home until the wee hours, but Lukasz would be. Lukasz, a Polish inventor, had come up with a revolutionary design for the aviation industry, a project I'd bought shares in. He used Dave's spare room as a workshop and it was good to finally meet him.

Day 15 | Wishaw to Crawford | 32.5 Miles

I woke up early as I could hear Dave mooching about downstairs.

'Chris, how you doing, man?' He beamed and gave me his usual bear hug.

'Fine, mate. Thanks for lending me your bed.'

Like a lot of people I'd met recently Dave seemed slightly confused by my charity endeavour, yet this didn't stop him accompanying me for three miles – after a bowl of porridge and a round of table football.

Following an early lunch of the 'haggis' I'd been looking forward to sampling since Angus Lennie played the irascible motel chef Shughie McFee in the hard-hitting soap

Crossroads, I found myself back in the Scottish countryside. As I ran along the rolling road into Lanark, fir trees gave way to deciduous forest on a landscape that could easily have been Devon. I crossed a tall bridge spanning a leafy river valley and began cruising up a hill so steep it would have crucified me as a young marine.

A chap stood leaning against the bonnet of his car wearing an expectant look behind a beard and glasses. 'Hello Chris!' He grinned. 'It's Johnny.'

'Whaaaat!'

Johnny had been a barman and me the doorman in Hong Kong's world-famous Rick's Café and I hadn't seen him for twenty-two years.

'I saw your Facebook post earlier and thought you must be on this road,' he said.

'Cup of tea?' I tendered.

'On me,' he replied and gave directions for the Petite Café.

Following our impromptu catch-up over a Rosy Lee I headed back into countryside that might well have been the Yorkshire Dales were it not for the occasional spruce plantation. True to her devious nature Sat Nav Woman began sending me up and down tiny roads, some of which appeared mere access tracks.

In the tiny village of Roberston I came across a chap in a beard unloading his car outside a white cottage.

'Where are you heading?' he asked.

'Land's End,' I puffed.

'Fancy a cup of tea?'

Legend!

'Andy' was a damn fine man and I thoroughly appreciated his north-of-the-border hospitality. He and his artist wife Poppy were a delightful couple and I left their brightly decorated bohemian home high on life, friendship and shortbread biscuits.

Approaching Abingdon I saw a sign declaring 'Gold panning in Scotland's highest village'. It didn't give the name of the village though, which was a real shame as I'd loved to have returned one day to strike it rich whilst ticking 'highest' off my bucket list.

I ducked into a Welcome Break petrol station, but with not a single meat-, egg- or cheese-free sandwich on offer I headed down the A702 – the main road into Carlisle before the M74 took all the glory – munching on a triple-decker sausage one. Had I a support team I would have asked them to prepare physically and mentally uplifting plant-based meals, but for speed and convenience I resolved to eat whatever lay at hand from this point forth.

It was dark now and I'd covered twenty-six miles. Not a single car passed me on this for-the-most-part-redundant highway, which explained why a lot of the roadside businesses had been boarded up. Trotting along I felt strangely out of place and unusually lonely and appreciated my 8pm call to Jenny and Harry all the more.

The traffic whizzing along the adjacent motorway wasn't helping my sense of unease. Knowing the drivers all sat in warm, coffee-cup-holding radio-blaring comfort and had a roof over their heads and family around them that night increased my feeling of being out on a limb. In addition the loud and constant hum of vehicle noise meant I couldn't pitch the tent for the foreseeable future.

After a further six miles the road veered away from its enthusiastic younger sibling and the Hungry Trucker Café appeared next to a vast and empty gravel-strewn lorry park. A sign told me I'd entered the village of Crawford, an eclectic mix of country homes, townhouses, old cottages and new-builds, clustered either side of a railway line – not that I had time to explore. A sudden downpour put paid to my aspirations of finding a pub for a late supper. I began exploring a patch of grass and nettles behind the café instead and the beam of my headlamp picked out of all things ... a *yurt*.

The yurt appeared to be a public attraction. With a slight tug I opened the unlocked door and peered inside. Reindeer skins lay on the yurt's octagonal bench and a medieval-looking fireplace sat in the centre. It was unlikely anyone would come here tonight, not in a full-on storm, and so I slipped inside. Fearing fleabites, I gave the stinky furs a miss and slept on the floor. I made sure to have my kit packed away by 6.30am to avoid a possible confrontation with Mongolian herders.

Day 16 | Crawford to Lockerbie | 32.3 Miles

After munching on a banana-and-raison-bread sandwich I ran seventeen miles along the deserted A702 into Beattock. Even though I needed the A7076 southbound towards Carlisle my brain got confused by a sign for the A701 and sent me east. Fortunately the miniature Silva compass clipped to my backpack strap showed me the error of my ways.

In the Old Stables pub I ate a vegetarian curry and *two* deserts while my sleeping bag dried in the sun. The girl serving behind the bar kindly pointed me in the right direction and I powered onwards, scrolling through my mobile to find the audiobooks and podcasts I'd copied – *in* a last-minute rush – to a specially bought 200 gigabyte memory card.

There was *nothing*.

All I could find in the phone's storage was Bill Bryson's *A Short History of Everything,* only it had uploaded to my phone in hundreds of mini-chapter files, none of which played in numerical order.

Plan B ...

As I attempted to access my online DropBox to download something else to occupy my ears the technological version of Groundhog Day kicked in and I stabbed at the touchscreen for twenty minutes before deciding to stick with my S Club 7, Boney M and Spice Girls classics.

A sign for Dumfries popped up. This surprised me as I would have placed such an iconic tartan name somewhere in the Highlands. After thirty-two miles I saw another unexpected sign, this time for Lockerbie. In an instant the carnage I'd witnessed in the media coverage of the Pan Am disaster came flooding back. In 1988 a bomb blew Flight 103 out of the sky and sent it crashing down on this unassuming town. Even though a pilgrimage to Lockerbie would add miles to my route, I felt I had to go there out of respect.

Jogging towards the town centre I couldn't recall the statistics – only that in addition to hundreds of passengers a number of residents had been killed and several houses demolished. The mere thought of the horror put my dicky knee and twinging quad muscle into perspective.

After my most-watched Facebook Live so far I entered the town pub to be greeted by the friendliest bar staff I'd ever met. My heart went out to these folks, their quiet little town forever synonymous with one of aviation's worst tragedies.

As I polished off a delicious vegetable stir fry with rice the landlord came over to suggest I pitch my tent in the town park. But worried about dog shit on the small square of grass I backtracked to Lockerbie's veterinary surgery and hopped over their fence into a field. Out of sight out of mind – not a bad tactic when you're camping.

Day 17 | Lockerbie to Carlisle | 32 Miles

I awoke in the usual swimming pool of sweat and condensation. Andy and Poppy had given me some fresh eggs and so I put them on to boil and commenced an Oscar-winning Facebook update. In the video, I took up my miniature camping towel and wiped a patch of the tent's flysheet, then squeezed half a cup of water out of the small cloth. I received a lot of well-meaning comments suggesting how I could waterproof the tent – but the problem originated inside not outside.

I didn't get on the road until midday having decided to visit the air disaster memorial garden. The date of the incident was 21st December, meaning the majority of the 279 passengers and crew would have been travelling home for Christmas, the eleven people killed in the town making preparations for the festive day. The memorial itself consisted of a polished-marble slab with the names of the dead etched into it.

Several plaques stood in memory to lost family members, one honouring a husband, a son *and* a daughter. Hard to imagine what that poor woman must have gone through. In an uplifting sentiment another tribute read 'Life is life. Enjoy it. Steven Lee Butler. 1952–1988'. It seemed strange to think Steven would have been sixty-six had he still been alive.

Back on the road, I passed a housing estate named in capitals: 'CLINT TERRACE' – and I'm sure I wasn't the only person that had to read that sign twice! My phone rang. It was Keith McLeod from Scotland's daily Record. We conducted an hour-long interview whilst I ran through the pouring rain.

Fifteen miles on I entered Gretna Green – another place I'd never planned to visit during my lifetime. My right quad muscle had been twitching and felt painful and mashed up below the skin and so I opted for some inexpensive on-the-spot therapy ... and ignored it.

Opposite the village sign stood a futuristic-looking hotel named Smiths. It's 'bar and restaurant' invitation was tempting but I continued forth to the Hazeldene Hotel, a mock-Tudor pub somewhat less snazzy than Smudger's grandiose gaff.

I sat in the Hazeldene enjoying gammon and chips with a bag of ice on my knee and two deserts on the way. My body craved the salt in the steak but I only ate half of it as too much animal protein would slow down my recovery time and give me a meat hangover. The door of the bar opened and in walked the enormous smile of Andrew Watson, an affable young reporter from a regional radio station. Andy oozed enthusiasm was extremely accommodating. *'No, no,* you *eat!'* he kept saying, clicking off his voice recorder in what had to be the most relaxed interview I'd ever done.

I picked up the pace along the B7076 and ran the remaining seventeen miles in one go because I was on my way to John 'Mac' McClelland in Carlisle. En route I passed the milestone that had been in my mind since embarking on the run – the 'Welcome to England' sign. With mixed emotions I took a selfie. I would miss Scotland and its wonderful people, who'd looked after me to an extent I'd never anticipated. All I could think was *Thank you.*

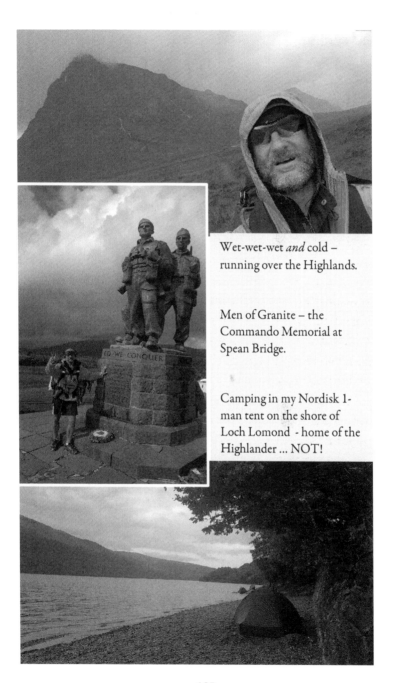

Wet-wet-wet *and* cold –
running over the Highlands.

Men of Granite – the
Commando Memorial at
Spean Bridge.

Camping in my Nordisk 1-
man tent on the shore of
Loch Lomond - home of the
Highlander ... NOT!

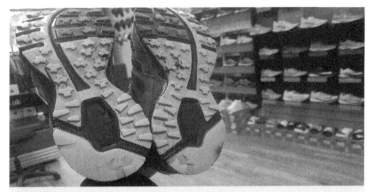

In Achilles Heel, Glasgow, for the first of four pairs of running shoes.

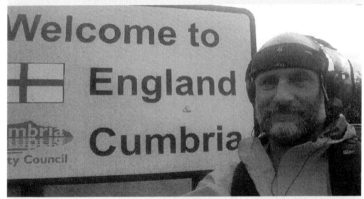

A great milestone.

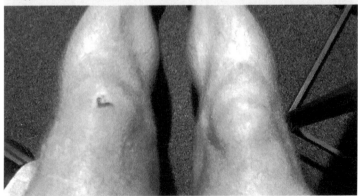

The right knee is mine – not sure about the left!

Fractured

Run rabbit, run rabbit, run run run.

Eminem

Day 18 | Carlisle to Shap | 31 Miles

Not surprisingly Mac was an absolute gentleman, a Royal Marines veteran who treated me like a son. In his modest suburban flat he cooked me an enormous plate of food and insisted I grab some kip in his bed. Whilst I slept this diamond of a man washed my clothes and dried my equipment. Before I left Mac looked me in the eye and said, 'Be *careful* over Shap!'

Following an early start I made Penrith by lunchtime. In the absence of any visible high-street eateries I ducked into the George Hotel, a grand redbrick building with an impressive Doric columned entrance. Ignoring the prices on the menu, I ordered a vegetable curry and charged my phone and iced my swollen knee while I ate. As with most days I had no destination in mind. A suitable camping spot usually dictated where I stopped.

Upon entering England I received an increasing number of requests for updates on my location and intended route. I'd been posting a picture of a UK map to my social media every night with a 'red line of progress' drawn on it – a screenshot taken from my sports tracker – as well as a daily mileage total. Now though, folks were asking me to be more precise so they could contemplate coming to support me.

The problem was I didn't have time to reply to anyone – I could read messages on the run but I couldn't hold the phone steady enough to write them – and I certainly wasn't going to start 'planning' or posting anything more than my current position and likely choice of road. In today's climate of rapid-fire of often thoughtless texting that would be inviting a liaison nightmare. And not only that but I didn't want the challenge to appear complex and put other people off achieving their dreams. As far as navigation was concerned I wanted folks to know that so long as your compass points south-*ish* and you've got a simple road map or a signal on your phone you're good to go.

Besides if folks were genuinely intent on supporting me they could plot roughly where I was from the updates or ask for my phone number. In the end I posted something along the lines of 'Left Carlisle at 7am and heading down the A6. With stops I average 4-5mph and so you can work out where I'll be.'

A break in the atrocious weather allowed me to enjoy the scenery all the more – for the most part rolling sheep fields and clusters of natural-stone farm buildings and old slate-tiled houses. The A6, the now quiet precursor to the M6, had a surprising amount of pavement along it for a country road. On the edge of Clifton the town's sign read 'Last Battlefield on English Soil. 1745' and featured a white rose with a black rose beneath it. I got the sneaking feeling the warring flowers had waited until I'd run past and then recommenced hacking the knobs off one another.

By now I'd jogged thirty miles and the breeze that had become a wind was now a storm, drowning out the *Born to Run* audiobook coming through my headphones. The tent could withstand 200kph gusts but the challenge lay in where to put it. Either side of the road were steep fields, which wasn't an issue in itself so long as I could find a suitably secluded corner. That way the field's drystone walls would afford some protection against the wind's constantly changing direction.

The problem was the gale blew with such force I'd have to close the zip on the tent to prevent the fabric from being ripped to shreds. My cramped quarters would become a vapour trap, soaking my clothing and sleeping bag once more and creating a potentially lethal situation what with the windchill.

It was cold now and I began to shiver. Stopping out in the open to put warm gear on would be inviting hypothermia and the clothing would only end up soaked by rain and sweat in minutes anyway. That lonely out-on-a-limb feeling returned with all its mates. What I would give to be in a nice warm hostel right now, diving into a camping saucepan full of backpackers' pasta whilst listening to round-the-world ticket holders announcing how they'd 'done' Machu Pichu. I needed shelter fast.

Growing ever more desperate I passed a small freight depot with parked-up lorries, stacks of pallets and an empty workers' caravan in it. *Should I see if the caravan is open?*

In the end I resolved to jog onwards, figuring like a *true* Englishman I should only resort to illegality after I'd actually frozen to death.

A sign appeared, 'Shap'. I remembered John mentioning this place – or had he *warned* me about it?

I fought off a crushing sense of disappointment. Not only would I have to continue for another couple of shivering miles to get through the village and find a place to camp but I'd also suffer the torment of passing houses boasting roaring fires, overflowing food cupboards *and* warm and dry duvets – and all for a night of cold clammy gale-force hell.

A turn-of-the-century row of terraced houses appeared – as did an enormous sheep shed and a smart barn conversion likely worth a fortune. A sign up ahead read 'New Ing Lodge' but seeing as though there are many different types of lodges – masonic, hunting and beaver for example – I didn't get too excited. A short but steep driveway led to what seemed to be a converted farmhouse, but even if this was a hostel there was no guarantee of a dormitory bed.

Daring to hope, I rang the bell ...

An athletic-looking young man wrenched the door open and grinned. 'Hi!'

'Hello mate. Is this a hostel?'

'It *certainly* is.'

'Have you got a room?'

'Dorm's empty so you've got it all to yourself. Fancy some broccoli soup and homemade bread?'

Some questions don't require an answer.

Day 19 | Shap to Carnforth | 33.81 Miles

After a delicious vegetarian breakfast, including the New Ing Lodge's speciality dish, 'green eggs', I conducted a stricter and more meticulous kit muster. The thirteen-kilo weight was running my body into the ground and I couldn't risk screwing up my ultramarathon-a-day average mileage and the chance to raise a decent sum for the Baton. It was time to implement my life-coaching strategy of having a Plan B that keeps Plan A on track – *and* jettison another kilo.

My stay at New Ing Lodge had been pure delight, literally the calm *during* a storm. Scott the hostel manager was an ultrarunner himself. As I settled my bill in the morning, he looked me warily in the eye. '*Good luck* over Shap.'

Heading for the village post office I thought nothing of it. I had more pressing issues on my mind. My knee was still blown up, the nape of my neck in agony from where the Y of the bergen straps constantly dug into it. To make matters worse the base of my battered spine kept sending me *Bugger!* messages.

'Thank you.' I handed the woman in the post office a parcel containing amongst other things the gas stove components and neoprene calf sleeves. The weighty sleeves made me sweat into my socks and I hadn't worn them since day two.

'Doing the Coast to Coast?' she asked, referring to the popular 192-mile horizontal trek across England.

'No, heading south,' I replied. 'Land's End.'

'Oh ...' The woman nodded thoughtfully – then *suddenly* fixed me with a beady satanic eye. '*Good luck* over Shap.'

For *heaven's* sake! It was starting to feel like the Slaughtered Lamb scene in *American Werewolf in London*. What the hell was it with this bloody Shap Fell? Didn't these children-of-the-corn types realise they were talking to a steely-eyed commando, one who'd crossed the Scottish Highlands in a pair of shorts ... and only had to be rescued *once*? How hard could a pancake-shaped challenge like Shap Fell be?

Putting it out of my mind I went outside and chucked my cooking pan and rations in a litter bin. Then I scrolled through the tracks on my MP3 player – Take That, Hoddle and Waddle, Saint Winifred's School Choir – before settling for Aqua's 'Barbie Girl' on *max* volume.

Everyone had warned me today's wind would be worse than yesterday and they weren't wrong. The problem was it blew in completely the wrong direction, making forward progress twice as hard – yet another scenario I hadn't envisaged while sipping umbrella drinks in the seaside paradise of Plymouth.

A car horn beeped in rapid succession. I looked up to see a male fist pump coming from a white car, followed by a champion wave. This was the second time my efforts had been acknowledged and my mood rocketed.

Once out of the village the A6 rose steeply. The houses gradually dropped away until there was only moorland, all of which appeared to be above me. Bang on cue the rain commenced, forcing me to duck into a pine plantation for fifteen minutes to avoid a soaking.

With my waterproof jacket on I continued upwards. The hill had become as steep as any I'd negotiated in the Highlands … but was *so* much longer. The mileage continued to accrue and I was *still* going up. At one point there was a cliff on the left-hand side of the road, a Rambo-like drop-off to right and no hard shoulder. Every time an oncoming vehicle approached I had to hop over the crash barrier and cling on for dear life.

As the significance of 'Good luck over Shap' finally sunk in I put some serious thought into my own safety. 'Exposed' didn't do my situation justice – 'madness' would be more accurate. Although not quite the cyclonic wind I'd experienced during Hong Kong's monsoon season it wasn't far off. At one point I couldn't make any headway into the gale and had to shelter behind a rocky outcrop until my wits and strength returned.

I began to consider turning around. Perhaps the occupants of the last farmhouse I passed would let me shelter until the worst of this was over. Two things went in my favour though – the occasional vehicle and the relatively mild temperature of the southerly blow.

Damn! I couldn't go backwards. Veterans were suffering and I had to go with my instincts and push on.

Upon reaching the summit I came across a stone hut named 'Shap Bothy'. What *perfect* timing and positioning! I'd read about these places. They'd provided refuge to shepherds in days gone by and now likewise to weary hikers – *free* of charge. With a sigh of relief, I launched a sopping-wet me through the door and into some sort of a vestibule.

I began stripping off my wet clothes.

'Errh …?' came a male voice.

I turned to see a guy peering through a gap in the doorway to the main room.

'Don't mind me, bud! I got *drenched* coming up the hill. Whack the kettle on, will ya?'

I pictured my intrepid adventuring self in a warm sleeping bag, propped against the shepherd hut's whitewashed walls, sipping chai while listening to the outrageous fell-related exploits of my fellow Shapsters.

The man continued to stare.

I noticed he wore smart slacks and a pinstriped office shirt. Something didn't feel right and so I peered past his torso to see an expensive-looking log burner roaring in the background. An elegantly-dressed wife-like person lounged on a spotless sheepskin rug next to a French-polished coffee table loaded with bottles of wine, crackers and huge slabs of yellow, orange and brown cheese. As for the romantic candles, I didn't know they were expecting me!

'Oh …' seemed a good place to start. 'I … *thought* this was a bothy?'

'It *is,*' the limited wardrobe replied.

This was confusing – perhaps Mr No Personality was a

mental head.

'No, I mean, I thought *anyone* could stay here?'

'They *could* in the past.'

The guy did 'stern' really well.

'But *this* one is *private* and *we're* on *holiday.*'

His partner grinned and fluttered her fingers.

'Well ...'

Come on Captain Clueless, at least offer me a hot drink. It's blowing a hooley out there!

'... I best be off then.'

Cursing Hospitality Henry for his city-slicking lack of humanity I ventured out into the storm. As I descended Shap's sissy profile and ran towards Kendall, clearing fallen tree branches out of the road as I went, I spotted the white car of earlier parked in a layby. 'John Capstick,' my fellow marine introduced himself. 'Thought you could do with a hotdog and a cup of coffee.' With a huge grin he handed me a Styrofoam cup.

I could have hugged the man – actually I did. What perfect timing and thoughtfulness. John said he was a driving instructor. He told me to stop in at Kendall Rugby Club, where a pint would be waiting for me on the bar.

Covering the last two of the sixteen miles into town I felt appreciated. News of my exploits had obviously travelled far and wide and I wondered if the whole of the rugby team would turn out to form a tunnel of respect and clap me in – or perhaps just the club's manager and apprentices.

By now the wind had dropped off and a luxurious strip of pavement led me along an enormous privet hedge, past several neatly mown pitches sprouting towering white Hs and into an entrance guarded by an electronic barber's-pole gate. Running towards the ultramodern clubhouse complex, I spotted a

Rhino Rugby scrummage machine in the training area. *I'll take it as a sign,* I thought, as my mum had once worked as a seamstress for Rhino.

There was none of the anticipated reception committee. *Probably getting ready to meet me in the bar ...*

I pictured a rowdy twelve-pint session culminating in me showing the boys how to shin up the goal posts naked and then them having a whip-round and chucking five-hundred quid into the charity pot and us all ending up in a tattoo parlour wearing misappropriated G-strings on our heads.

I entered the smart reception and wafted a flamboyant 'Hi!' to the smartly dressed young woman behind the desk. I chucked in an A-lister smile so she knew I was 'the guy'.

'Upstairs.' She pointed and gave me a cheeky grin.

Having straightened my bandana before meeting the team, I entered the plush bar to find ... *no one.*

Huh?

A bartender stared into a bowl of peanuts.

As my short-lived celebrity crashed to the floor, 'Hello mate,' I said. 'I'm here for my complimentary pint – but can I have a cuppa instead?'

'Sorry?' the young man replied, looking at me askance.

'I'm Chris. The guy who's running the length of the country. Apparently there's a drink here waiting for me.'

'It's the first I've heard of it.' The barman shrugged. 'But you deserve that cuppa.'

Day 20 | Carnforth to Bilsborrow | 24.7 Miles

At the ten-mile point the next morning I realised I had a problem. The iliotibial or 'IT' bands running down the outside of my knees had flared up again. This first happened last night. A former Royal Marine turned recovery truck firm operator Alistair and his caring wife Sarah had invited me to stay with them at their stunning barn conversion in Carnforth. Following Android Navigator's instructions, which had taken me down quiet back lanes, I'd pushed the miles up to thirty-four, looking forward to our rendezvous. After a while though this increasingly intense pain set in. Every three hundred metres I'd had to stop and massage my inflamed tendons in order to continue.

Al had introduced me to a TENS or 'Transcutaneous Electrical Nerve Stimulation' machine, basically a pulsating current that flows between two sticky pads to massage your sore areas. I bore the stabbing electric shocks to my spasming leg muscles with stoicism, only it didn't help my shredded IT bands. The extremely hospitable former marine also offered to post the three-seasons sleeping bag home as Brommers had arranged for Jenny to send my much lighter Mammut one to Cath Green, whose family I'd be staying with tomorrow night. This would shed half a kilo in weight and hopefully stop me sweating so much.

En route to Al and Sarah's I'd stopped to check directions outside the Longlands Hotel, a majestic white pub flying hanging baskets and the flags of all nations. A white van driver beeped his horn and screeched to a halt in front of me.

I tensed up thinking this guy might well be another Great British drama queen who'd yet to suss the brake pedal or work out what a steering wheel is.

The man jumped out of the vehicle and waggled an accusatory finger at me. 'You're *that* guy!'

'Which guy?' I tendered, wondering if he referred to the proud owner of no less than *four* 1000-piece jigsaw puzzles.

'The guy on *Facebook!*' He beamed. 'Who's *running* the

length of the country!'

Wow! I pictured myself drowning in silicon and suntan oil on *Celebrity Love Island*.

Today I was heading for 'Dolly' Dolman's place in Bamber Bridge, thirty-three miles away. By staying with the former bootneck tonight I didn't have to worry about not having a sleeping bag until tomorrow. If I had more miles in my legs upon reaching Bamber Bridge I would continue down the A6 until exhausted and Dolly would come and pick me up. If people wanted to support me it was appreciated but I'd made it clear to Brommers that they had to respect my ultramarathon-a-day average.

In the pouring rain I was struggling to make the distance. My IT bands were beyond torture and I'd developed a sore spot on my lower shin. I put on a tubular ankle support but it only made the pain worse. Dolly called wanting to know where to pick me up. 'I'm *not* ready yet mate,' I told him, determined to crack at least a marathon.

The great thing about being in Lancashire and passing through so many towns and villages was the liberal sprinkling of petrol stations and convenience shops. I no longer had to waste precious time waiting to be served in pubs. My diet took an unavoidable downturn though and now consisted of sandwiches, slices, chocolate, crisps and the occasional Cherry Coca-Cola. I wasn't too bothered. My muscles needed the calories and I would arrive at Land's End with my ultras in the bag no matter what.

Dolly called again and I let slip I had a stress fracture, known in the military as a 'shin splint'. Every time I planted my right foot it felt as if someone had shoved a spear through my lower leg. 'I'm fine though, Dolls, honest.'

'I'm coming to get you!' Dolly argued.

The pain grew worse because I was forced to increase the pace in an attempt to make marathon distance before the day got cut short.

A white transit pulled into a layby up ahead. 'Chris!' the driver greeted me from his open window. 'I'm Andy. My buddy's an ex-bootneck and he sent me to check you're alright.'

I hopped into the passenger seat for a hug and a cup of coffee from the thermos Andy had thoughtfully brought. After a brief chat I got back on the road, conscious of having to knock off four miles to achieve ultramarathon status. Andy insisted on driving ahead and waiting for me to run past, which was touching.

Dolly pulled up in a sleek-lined mid-life crisis and I reluctantly lowered my aching body down to a height appropriate for boy racers and four-year-olds. 'Come on mate, let's get you in the bath.'

'Erh ...' My fractured shinbone really needed ice but now the seed had been planted a hot soak was too hard to resist.

'Do you fancy Indian or Chinese?'

'Just a plate of vegetables please Dolls,' I replied.

It was imperative I purge the acid building up in my tissues from all the service station crap I'd funnelled down my neck. I didn't want to risk getting ill for the first time in years and seriously screwing things up.

'*Vegetables?*' Dolls frowned.

'Yeah – like carrots.'

'*Carrots?*'

'Orange things, grow in the mud, rabbits love 'em.'

'Right ...' Dolly murmured, looking utterly bewildered. 'So ... *chicken* stir fry, you mean?'

'Nah, *just* vegetables, mate.' I chuckled. '*Please.*'

'Okay ...' Dolls nodded thoughtfully. 'We'll go for *pork* then.'

Day 21 | Bilsborrow to Bamber Bridge | 12.6 Miles

At breakfast Doll's doting wife Jaki gave me a card and a bowl of porridge.

Upon opening the card I realised it was my birthday. Now, should I take the day off or run an ultramarathon with a broken leg?

Decisions ...

As Dolly drove us back to the place he'd picked me up a former Royal Marine turned physio, Harry Black, gave me advice over the phone. It was truly appreciated but the amount of pain I was in and the bloody bruise ringing my shin told me this wasn't going to be fixed with ibuprofen and a tennis ball massage. Oh well, I'd run the five-hundred miles to Land's End with a fractured limb – *end of.*

'Running' turned out to be a slightly ambitious term. I *could* run – only it was so much agony I worried my tibia would snap completely and I'd have to waste time getting a plaster cast in A&E before continuing. Instead I adopted a kind of leg-vaulting hobble, projecting the sort of image that makes cage fighters cross the road to avoid you.

By eight in the evening I'd limped for fourteen hours and managed less than thirteen miles. Dolly pulled up in the Batmobile. 'How you doing, Royal?' he asked.

'Leg's a bit sore but I'm fine, bro,' I lied.

'Come back and stay another night. I'll get you a bag of ice.'

My shin needed some proper rest and *I* needed to figure a way to keep heading south. Accepting Dolly's offer seemed the best course of action.

Another former marine turned up at the house. Jason Wilcock was a chap I'd served with in 42 Commando. We'd undergone Arctic warfare and survival training in Norway together and fought in the Northern Ireland Conflict. 'J' was a cracking professional photographer with a personality to match. He immediately sat me down for a strategy meeting. 'If you can't run you'll have to continue limping.' He nodded my agreement. 'Setting off dead early and continuing until midnight to get the ultra.'

'Yep ... yep ...' My brain ran through the time versus distance calculation. It felt great to have a workable Plan B.

While I sat with my leg iced and elevated J and Dolly celebrated my birthday, necking Stella Artois as if someone was going to steal it. It was rewarding to see two strangers crack on like long-lost brothers – something perhaps only a Royal Marine can understand. I didn't miss the booze – not even on my birthday. When you break a habit for ninety days – almost two years in my case – the allure evaporates and it ceases to have any sort of hold over you.

Day 22 | Bamber Bridge to Wigan | 14.3 Miles

Despite their banging beer heads the boys were up at 5am, as was Jaki, to get me on the road. I ate a bowl of porridge and then J took some shots of us all with his state-of-the-art gear. J and I said goodbye to our wonderful hosts and drove back to the point I'd reached the day before.

Having taken the day off work to support me J disappeared every so often to grab food and medical supplies. He even managed to arrange a complimentary meal in the Boar's Head and a generous donation from the landlady. I scraped fourteen miles into Wigan, albeit at a quicker pace than yesterday, J keeping me focused and attending to my every need. Worryingly though, the pain had increased. It was time to stop putting stress on the fracture and so I reluctantly called Brommers to find out where I'd be staying tonight.

Cath Green and her husband Tim and two daughters were wonderful individuals. They welcomed me with open arms *and* a birthday cake decorated with my #999miles Facebook banner. My lightweight sleeping bag had arrived too, shedding another kilo of burden. Over a delicious chicken dinner I got to know Cath's friend James Harrington, a former Royal Marines medic with tours of Afghanistan under his belt.

'Rest and ice, Chris,' James urged. 'The ice constricts the area and then as the tissue rewarms it draws in fresh blood to help to mend the wound.'

I decided to test the leg in the morning – thus ticking the box for not taking a day off. If I sensed the pain getting worse and undoing all of the precious healing I would rest for the afternoon and evening. This would add four miles a day to my future-required tally, meaning I'd have to average at least thirty-two miles every twenty-four hours, *with* a broken leg, for the next fortnight. It was a gamble but I had no other choice ...

Day 23 | Wigan | 0.47 Miles

Half a mile into the twenty-third day I could tell my leg was attempting to heal but one wrong footfall would put me immediately back to square one. By sticking to my plan to rest for the remainder of the day, I stood a chance of keeping my ultra dream alive. I sat in the sun outside a Tesco and announced my intentions on social media, before calling Cath and Tim.

Then I saw a sight that fell somewhere between bizarre and strange – a man cycling down the road in a ... *bath!* I had the honour of flagging down Britain's most dedicated fundraiser Stuart 'the Mad Fool' Kettell, whose outrageous efforts for the Macmillan charity had seen him push a sprout up Mount Snowden with his nose and run seven marathons inside a gigantic hamster wheel whilst dressed as one of the rodents.

'How's it going?' I asked Stu, who'd dyed his Keith-Flint-style hair fluorescent green for the occasion.

'Got a sore ass, mate.' He grimaced.

I peered into the tub to see his sole cushion consisted of a rubber bath mat. What a trouper!

My stay at Cath and Tim's place would have bordered on majestic were it not for having to run a further 450 miles with a fractured shin. All I could do was rest, ice and visualise reaching Land's End.

While sitting on the couch in the front room, blanking out Sky's fake news flickering on the widescreen, I got a message from my friend Katie. She'd sent me a full-page article the *Plymouth Herald* had run on my JOGLE story. I had to smile. Along with using *my* photos, they'd simply transcribed my Facebook JOGLE information video word for word – talk about *lazy* journalism!

The Greens were a super family and their genuine hospitality *and* Cath's reiki massage were exactly what I'd needed at this moment in time. It was emotional having to say goodbye to them.

Pirate

Run really fast.

Nigel Mansell

Day 24 | Wigan to Tarporley | 31.29 Miles

The sun shone on my face – nature's way of letting me know I was alright. My shin was fine ... *for* the first ten miles, but by the time I reached Warrington the full extent of the pain had come flooding back. I returned to my woeful limp, grimacing as I passed lines of cars waiting at traffic lights, their drivers staring at me in bemusement. Yet it was no good. My heart told me I was never going to make the ultramarathon distance.

Desperate times call for desperate measures. On the edge of Warrington I unstrapped my backpack and sank down on the pavement outside a sports hall, resigning myself to yet another Plan B to support Plan A – painkillers. I hadn't popped any until now as I didn't want to risk lulling myself into a false sense of security and worsening the damage to my leg. In order to continue though, I had no choice and necked two pills.

I bought ice and some nappy bags in a Lidl. Then using my bandana I strapped a bag with about ten frozen cubes in it around my shin. The combination of cold and meds made an enormous difference and before long I was running past the Tim Parry and Johnathan Ball memorial in the centre of town.

From Warrington I ran along the River Mersey, shirtless, soaking up the rays and loving my newfound respite from the pain. I crossed the Manchester Ship Canal and then queued for the swing bridge over the River Weaver at Acton before continuing towards a place called Tarporley.

The pain relief changed my outlook on life and I made the next Facebook broadcast with a traffic cone on my head. As I continued along the A49 a white van pulled alongside and its driver shouted, 'Are you *homeless,* mate?'

'Yes,' I replied truthfully.

The sound of a bike engine caught my attention and I turned to see James Harrington pulling up. What a kind man and a true brother, driving a fifty-mile round trip just for a two-minute chat to check I was okay.

Helen 'Sweeney' Todd, a former Wren turned sports scientist, got in contact to offer me physio treatment and a bed for the night. But as I sat in a café charging my phone and nursing a cuppa, I worked out she lived too far off my route.

Darkness drew in and I had no idea where I would stop for the evening. I'd run through Scotland not realising you can camp pretty much anywhere. However, I was in the totalitarian state of England now, where eating McDonald's is promoted on television but teaching your kids about the Great Outdoors is taboo. It sounds unbelievable in a country responsible for the most rough-sleepers in Europe – not that I had a problem breaking this particular law.

My issue lay in the lie of the land itself. As I trotted along Tarporley Road thick hedgerows sprouted sturdy native trees either side of me. Every gap I glanced through revealed some form of private property – vegetable fields, poly tunnels, stables, lavish country homes, sports pitches – plus there was the traffic noise to get away from. I wasn't sure at which point I should go off road to look for a suitable spot. I didn't want to cut my day unnecessarily short nor did I want to end up struggling along exhausted and wishing I'd staked my claim earlier.

There was a white Ford Fiesta parked on the pavement ahead. A thick-set chap and a young girl leant against its bumper. 'Hello, Chris.' The guy put his hand out. 'Neil Davies – former bootneck – and this is Drew. Heard you needed some ice.'

Neil told me he'd spent eight years in Corps and had driven several miles from Flint to meet up with me. He loaded me up with ice, a Lucozade and a ham-and-cheese roll and invited me to stay with them tonight. For the second time today I had to decline such a thoughtful offer, Neil's place being way off my path. I didn't mind. I liked sleeping in the tent and now that I had the lighter sleeping bag perhaps my night would be a lot less sweaty and not as cold.

After running along telling Harry a story about philanthropic eagles bigger than houses, I ducked down a leafy lane and began searching for a sleeping spot. But there was nothing suitable – only fields in direct line of sight of their owner's properties, most appearing to have some sort of connection to equestrian activities.

I resorted to crossing four fields in an attempt to become anonymous. Having crawled through a barbed-wire fence, I found myself standing in the pitch black on a surprisingly *flat* field. If I set up my tent by one particularly thick part of the boundary hedge several other hedgerows aligned to block out all of the lights from surrounding premises – the logic being the owners wouldn't be able to see mine. I scoffed an egg sandwich, wrapped my smock around the wafer-thin sleeping bag and had a deep *and* dry night's sleep – despite my phone showing it had been minus *three!*

Day 25 | Tarporley to Prees Green | 31 Miles

I packed up early as the sun began to burn away the dappled-red clouds overhead. Only then did I discover the reason behind the flatness under foot – I'd slept on a *polo field!*

Four miles south on the A49 I came across a somewhat unique venture – the Red Fox *Indian* Restaurant. Amazed to find it open at this up-and-at-'em hour I decided to make a breakfast stop, sitting down at a cream tablecloth to ponder vindaloo or rogan josh.

No one appeared and so I rang the bell on the bar.

Following a sound like an elephant playing the drums with a kettlebell a middle-aged Indian chap crashed through the nearest door in his boxer shorts. He looked at me sideways.

'I suppose onion bhaji's are out of the question?' I shrugged.

'Six o'clock tonight, sir,' the gentleman replied through a yawn.

'In that case can I get some ice instead, please?'

The grey-haired proprietor gave me so much of the cold stuff I had to throw half of it away. Despite its slack approach to security if you ever need the authentic flavour of India while smashing out a pub quiz then the Red Fox in Tarporley is the place for you.

An English-heritage sign caught my attention. I smiled. 'Beeston Castle' was a place my late mate Lee had loved to spend time. He'd go there with his mates after visiting hours and they'd pop pills and wander around the grounds off their heads. For Lee's funeral everyone partied for forty-eight hours and then took it in turns to throw a handful of his ashes off the ramparts.

I wandered along contented, enjoying a rolling agricultural landscape dotted with enormous oaks. The pavement accompanying this stretch of country road was set five-metres back from the traffic and shaded by tall drooping willows. Sunlight mottling on my face sent me into a dream world. I was in heaven and it was brilli –

The Armed Response Unit *screeched* to a halt in front of me …

An officer climbed from his vehicle and motioned me to stop …

I froze on the pavement …

… Actually it *was* a member of the police's elite firearms unit, only he was clad in stretchy black man-gear and cycling shoes – as opposed to Kevlar and an MP5. Pushing his racing bike across the grass verge, 'Fish!' The six-foot-three chap put his hand out.

Nah, I'm okay thanks.

'They called me fish in the Marines because I was good at swimming,' Mathew 'Fish' Peterson continued.

Matt was an absolute diamond and a great example of the down-to-earth and personable characters the Royal Marines recruits. Considering I hadn't felt the need for company so far on my jaunt I thoroughly enjoyed our time together. We chatted about all sorts of things while negotiating the A9's winding lanes. The treacherous traffic on the blind bends forced us to come to an arrangement with respect to crossing the road – namely that we would both do our own thing and dash across when the time was right. This avoided confusion and the potential to get each other run over – especially as Fish had the added responsibility of pushing his racing bike. Fish bought me … *fish* pie for lunch at the Cholmondeley Arms and a coffee at Starbucks, where I tasked him with the day's Facebook video update.

Continuing forth I headed for Russell Humphrey's place in Shrewsbury. I hadn't met Russ before but he was a dedicated part of a growing movement named Veterans United Against Suicide. A mutual friend Davey Robb, the youngest marine to have served in the Falklands Conflict, had put us in touch.

I had a problem though. Despite me doubling the dose of ibuprofen and continuing with the painkillers my fractured leg was agony beyond belief – so too the IT bands where they passed the outsides of my knees. Slowing down wasn't an option or I wouldn't make the ultramarathon distance. I had to power through the intense pain, which meant stopping every five-hundred metres to massage my knees and reapply ice.

Davy called to say he was at Russ's and they were coming to pick me up.

'No, *please* don't!' I yelled over the traffic noise. 'I'll call you when I'm done.'

As a result of that half a day of rest in Wigan I *had* to run a minimum of thirty-three miles a day to Land's End. This would keep my ultramarathon-a-day on target and I was sticking to it no matter what. I'd covered another ten miles since leaving Fish and now had over thirty clocked up on the Endomondo app. If I ran the thirteen miles into Shrewsbury it would significantly improve my statistics and the chance of success. I turned on my flashing hazard lights and continued on around the dark bends.

Fortunately the pain had no chance of affecting my mood. So focused on raising awareness of veterans' mental health I ignored the excruciating discomfort. My sole concern was keeping my body functioning long enough to reach Cornwall. Davy rang again asking for a location so he could come and get me. 'I'm *not* finished mate,' I puffed. 'I'll bell you.'

Twenty minutes later a shiny white VW Golf came hammering around a corner. It screeched to a stop and two burly ex-marines leapt out and bundled me inside.

Talk about your wildest fantasy coming true!

Day 26 | Prees Green to Church Stretton | 32.24 Miles

Russ was your archetypal well-built, strong-jawed and modest firefighter, a guy who projected the sort of cool calm confidence you'd pray for when trapped in a burning building. His place was immaculate and the salmon he cooked for the three of us delicious. Both he and Davy were Class of 82 Falklands veterans. Davy tucked twenty quid in my hand for expenses and coached me through some serious stretching exercises – ones he'd learned while boxing for the Corps. Then with a Veterans United Against Suicide band on my wrist we set about taking photos and making a video speech with the organisation's flag as a backdrop.

In the morning I checked the charity total and was amazed to see it hovering above the seven thousand pounds mark. Baz had reckoned the majority of money would come in on the last day, which was reason alone to reach Land's End – not that I needed additional incentive. Two years ago I'd made my mind up to complete the JOGLE and now all I had to do was put in the legwork.

I continued to post to the Facebook page a UK map with the red line of progress drawn on it. Each day it produced increasing amazement. 'Wow, you're *halfway* down Wales already!' exclaimed one geographer. 'Gosh, I thought you were still in Scotland,' wrote another. But the best comments were along the lines of, *'Bloody hell,* you're almost at Land's End!'

Having loaded me up with water and snacks Russ drove us back to the roadside. I was running along listening to my tunes and not investing too much thought into the changing vista, but if forced to describe it I'd probably say something about a green and pleasant land and hop into a Spitfire. The well-manicured hedgerows, pristine liquorice-black tarmac, smart stone walls, ye-olde pubs and impressive mix of ancient and new housing hinted you needed a few bob in your pocket to live around these parts.

As midday arrived a powerful motorcycle pulled up behind me.

'Nice bike, mate.'

'Cheers Chris.' Russ removed his helmet and patted the BMW tourer's chunky leather seat. 'My new hobby.'

Russ caught up with me twice more before I left the Shrewsbury area and when we finally said goodbye I couldn't have been better looked after.

Today was hard going. The pain from my fractured leg and damaged IT bands was now so severe it rose above the threshold of the morning's painkillers. I took a second dose … to no avail. I hobbled along wincing yet making steady progress, only the increasing agony told me this wasn't sustainable. If I didn't come up with a Plan B sharpish I'd have to admit defeat on my ultramarathon-a-day average and go home.

A horn beeped as a car stopped on the verge. A clean-cut athletic-looking young man hopped out wearing a military flight suit. 'Jay Whitehouse, Chris. Former marine turned aircrew.' He shoved his hand out. 'What can I get you?'

Jay had recognised me from the Facebook page and wanted to check I was okay. When I told him about my spaghetti legs and mashed potato knees he said, 'Have you thought about walking poles?'

The boys I'd met on the first day had asked me the same question. I'd never given them serious consideration because I didn't particularly like the idea of 'walking' *and* carrying extra equipment for the privilege. I'd seen people using walking poles on ultras and they just looked like a truckload of hassle. 'I guess it might relieve some of the stress on my injuries.' I nodded, running short of options.

A couple of hours later Jay returned and handed me an extendable pole. 'Sorry it's only one.' He shrugged. 'But I'm working on getting another.'

Eyeing the sole pole I had an image of Jay running door to door in his village begging pensioners to donate their disability aids to the cause. We agreed I would message him the location of my tent that evening. Ten minutes later another Facebook supporter's car skidded to a halt in a layby. A fellow veteran Emma Kay hopped out, gave me a huge hug and made a generous donation the next day.

I struggled onwards checking replies to my last Facebook update in which I'd mentioned I was travelling down the A49 towards Hereford, home of Britain's elite Special Air Service. But it was no good. I made it to the village of Dorrington and collapsed on a grassy bank out front of The Old Hall, a majestic Tudor former pub offering 'Persian Cuisine – Shropshire's First!'

I would have laughed ... only I was too preoccupied with the distinct reality my mission was about to end if I didn't come up with a plan *el rapido*. There was no way I was cutting down the daily mileage *or* resting *or* walking to Land's End.

... And yet there was no way I could continue. It wasn't that I couldn't *run* – it was that I could no longer *walk*. The agony in my knees and fractured leg matched that of my tortured head. My dream stood in tatters, shot out of the sky like a flock of angels blasted by a toff with a twelve bore. The words of my recruit buddy Colin echoed in my mind: 'If you pull this off, Chris, you can dine out on it for life.'

He was right – only failure meant *so* much more. My anticipated career progression – namely the ability to support and inspire others *and* cover my modest outgoings – would take a serious hit. Plus there was the time, money and energy Jenny and I had invested. I was two thirds of the way down the country, having survived a fortnight of atrocious weather. *Damn,* I was *almost* there! It would be a huge hassle to have to go through all of this again.

I *couldn't* stop ...

I *wouldn't* stop ...

My back was against the wall, way past the point where most people would have admitted defeat and gone home. But there's *always* a way ... and a tot of rum might just numb the pain enough for me to grit my teeth and continue.

Hadn't I run past a Premier shop and don't they sell booze?

Backtracking to the off licence I negotiated a new intrusion on my mood. During twenty-four alcohol-free months my life had flown ten miles above brilliant, my relationships solid, my early mornings hangover-free, productive and spiritually fulfilling.

I wasn't overly concerned about the addictive effect of alcohol – I knew my own strength of mind – but like a cricketer who'd experienced an unbroken run of centuries it was deeply disappointing having to voluntarily bow out.

I entered the Premier shop and bought a small bottle of

pirate juice. Then I sat on the bank outside Shropshire's *first* Persian restaurant and took a slug. Within seconds my destiny had changed and I was flying along the country lanes.

The dream was back on!

Buster

Don't stop the body rock.

Fu Manchu

Day 27 | Church Stretton to Leominster | 26.81 Miles

'Morning, mate!' Jay grinned, waggling a walking pole at me. 'Got your other stick.'

'Well done brother!' I peeled the tent flap back to a more sociable angle.

'Bought you some snacks as well.' He dumped a veritable supermarket sweep onto the grass.

'Cheers dude. Don't think me rude if I don't take all of them. I've got to keep the weight off my shin splint.'

Jay was fine about it and after a hug I got under way towards Ludlow. Last night I'd treated myself to a pub dinner and a pint of real ale in the Buck's Head, then found a perfect camping spot behind the local church.

Despite a morning slug of rum the pain returned immediately. While testing out the walking poles I wracked my mind for a Plan C that wouldn't screw up Plan A.

First off, these hikers' sticks could go to a new home. I was extremely grateful to Jay, only the poles were more hindrance than help. Perhaps negotiating steep rocky trails I would have got some benefit from them. Along the relatively flat tarmac though, they served no function – other than to weigh an additional half-kilo.

With another ten days or more to reach Land's End it was time to pull out all the stops. I needed to go rogue and ditch the poles along with every last gram of unnecessary weight. I sat under a tree on a neatly mown patch of grass outside a stately home and conducted yet another full kit muster.

My already tiny wash kit and small square of towel could go. I'd have to grab a quick splash in service stations and rivers where possible. The sterilisation tablets and first-aid kit were also history. I'd keep the painkillers and ibuprofen, so too the large oval-shaped blister plasters – I needed one now. Running with a limp for hundreds of miles had caused my right heel to rub and I could no longer ignore it. My remaining T-shirt had already gone into Room 101 – I'd been wearing my smock during the cool evenings and nothing during the day. Four pairs of socks followed suit, leaving me two. My small lightweight pillow went to the big bed in the sky – my smock would have to do now. A small screw-top pot of sun cream remained unused. I had a slightly red nose as a result of the glare from my shades, but not enough of a problem to warrant carrying fifty surplus grams.

In total I kept my mobile phone, MP3 player and headphones, triple-USB fast-charger, sunglasses, bandana, smock, shorts, the socks, my trainers, bergen, bum bag, tent, sleeping bag and inflatable mat, flashing lights and headtorch, broken-body meds, a couple of blister plasters, the rum, waterproof trousers and jacket. I clipped the now-redundant stuff sack for my clothes onto the waist strap of my rucksack to hold the bags of ice I bought.

Although I'd managed to get my kit down to around ten kilos it was still the weight of a large microwave oven – and try hefting one of those a thousand miles! I shoved the redundant gear into a litterbin by the entrance of the National Trust's open-to-the-public mansion and balanced the walking poles on top so hopefully someone could put them to good use.

Approaching Ludlow I recognised a face I hadn't seen since school. Karen Down stood at the side of a forest road waiting to greet me. As if this wasn't fantastic in itself, my old friend had bought me a bag of ice *and* an enormous tray of sushi!

'It's amazing what you're doing,' Karen kept saying, making my efforts feel appreciated. 'You're in *so* much pain and you *keep* going!'

'I don't know what to say.' I shrugged. 'I just head south.'

Karen had bought me a stack of food and drinks. I packed a day's worth into the side pocket of my bergen and filled the stuff sack with ice. All too soon we were saying goodbye.

Ludlow was harmless enough for Little England – only the poor town had no idea what year it was. Tudor timbers jostled for exposure with medieval granite, latter-day red bricks and Plain-Jane frontages from god knows what period. Not that I was taking much in. The unrelenting pain meant all I could think about was putting one blistered foot in front of the other in a single-minded effort to get the mileage done.

'Chris!' came a voice from behind.

I turned to see Matt, a good-natured chap who'd said hello to me as I approached the town and asked what gives. He must have jumped in his car to catch me up.

'I want to help.' He looked at me in earnest.

'Nice one, Matt. Could you share my Facebook posts –?'

'*No* – I mean I want to help you financially – with food, equipment, *anything.*'

I thought hard. 'Some new insoles? My injuries are pretty bad now.'

Matt chaperoned me to the nearest pharmacy, but when I saw the price of their gel inserts – *thirty-five* quid – I felt embarrassed.

'Matt, don't worry. I'll be fine.'

'*No!* I want to help you.' The legend pulled out his wallet.

The new shock absorbers worked a treat and stayed with me until Land's End – as did Matt's generosity and human kindness.

I left 'Probably the loveliest town in England' (as described by Sir John 'Sit on the Fence' Betjeman) on the B4361 and crossed the River Teme courtesy of an immaculately restored single-lane stone bridge. At the end of the ancient span ensconced the Charlton Arms. The listed building's period appearance accommodated three fantastic terraces majestically shrouded in trademark English greenery, each level enjoying an exquisite view out over the meandering Teme's oily olive waters. It had to be one of the most unique boozers on the planet – not that I had time for a pint.

While making the most of the pavement before hitting the less friendly A49 it occurred to me I hadn't much battery on the phone. Wanting to keep my tracker running I entered Overton Petrol Station and asked the grey-haired owner if I could plug in. 'Sure,' he replied. 'Fancy a cuppa?'

'Thanks very much!' I beamed, visualising this much-welcomed bonus.

'Back in a minute.' He wandered off the forecourt.

Twenty minutes later my phone had a seventy percent charge. Lord Lucan had yet to return with my char and so I unplugged from the mother ship and slipped moorings. I felt a bit rude. Perhaps the gentleman was still waiting for the kettle to boil. If so, he needed a new one.

On the charity page I was honoured to find Facebook's 'speshul' forces comedy legend Dirk Steel and his 'useless' hound Colin had donated two hundred pounds. Dirk's kind gesture kept my mood up no end, but on the downside my companion named Pain meant I'd covered pitiful few miles this day and still had another fifteen or more to do. It was time to *man ... woman ...* or *person* up and get today's ultra in the bag.

My problem was the killer traffic on the A49 – today's oncoming culprits forming a particularly bad flow of visually challenged double-handcuffed swine – *and* it was getting dark. Having hurdled a marrow, I came upon a Travel Lodge and stopped to stare through the lounge bar window, taking in flaccid-bellied business reps, white shirts open at the collar, tucking into mouth-watering plates of grub.

Forget the injuries, this was my *toughest* dilemma so far. *Should I ...?* I asked myself, picturing bangers and mash, a golden pint and spotless linen. The lonely, cold and out-on-a-limb feeling returned as juggernauts thundered past me like props in a *Mad Max* film. Upon spotting my flashing lights and reflective fluorescent-striped jacket, idiot car drivers had insisted on blaring their horns, leaving me no option but to hop onto the clumpy grass verge. I'd been forced to put my headtorch on to avoid – unsuccessfully – falling down numerous holes.

Should I could cut today's mileage short and treat myself to a night in the Travel Lodge?

It was *so* tempting, but I knew I had a job to do. I returned to the verge and stumbled forth into the darkness.

With my ultramarathon mileage completed I stopped in a layby outside Leominster to get my bearings. Exhausted, I wondered whether to continue past the town before searching for a camp spot.

'What are you doing?'

I turned to see a chap standing by a smart campervan and

smoking a ciggie. 'Just figuring a place to stay,' I replied.

'Fancy a cuppa?' He smiled. 'I'm Dale.'

Dale ushered me inside the mobile home and introduced me to his partner Steve and their two poodles. After a brew the wonderful chaps invited me to crash. Lying in duvet heaven on an extremely comfortable double bed, *Who needs a Travel Lodge?* I thought.

Day 28 | Leominster to Three Ashes | 30 Miles

Steve was so moved by my efforts he decided to follow in my footsteps and attempt the JOGLE the coming year. The boys filled me with tea and toast and after hugs all round I struck out for Hereford, looking forward to my hero's welcome with the Special Air Service. I could picture it now – Mandy Kebab and his desert daredevils clapping wildly and shouting 'Welcome *home,* brother! *Three* cheers for the *Regiment!*' – me entering my spiritual home to take up my honorary place 'on the Balcony'.

Oh yes, it's a life of storming Bahrainian embassies and tipping scorpions out of my boots for me!

I craned around the next corner, looking forwards to catching a glimpse of Dirk Steel and the rest of my special forces reception committee.

There was *no one* ... except a member of the Royal Marines' elite Special Boat Service, the 'SBS'.

John Nash was an old oppo of mine from recruit training. In military circles it's generally accepted that our 'Fighting 558 Troop' consisted of the hardest and most handsome rogues ever to grace camouflage – and who am I to disagree? John Nash, with his tight pink shorts, Magnum P.I. chest rug, whopping great gold chains and hoop earrings, personified this dashing derring-do-ness, taking macho to a whole new level – as did his pit-bull terrier Tyson and the enormous key chain jangling from his belt. Every man wanted to be like John ... and so did a lot of women.

His state-of-the-art truck sat in the entrance of a farmer's field. 'Where've you been, you *ninja* turtle?' He grinned, chuckling at my dayglow green backpack cover.

'*Fucked,* mate. Fell asleep in a corn field.'

'Well, there's a Beefeater just up the road, boyo. I'll see you in there – scran's on me.'

John had undoubtedly been the fittest member of our troop, hardly surprising as the stocky six-footer had played youth rugby for Wales. Having left the special forces, John had gone on to become one of the country's most successful business persons *and* a world-renowned ballet coach. It was wonderful to see him and wolf down a vegetable curry before getting treated to a new pair of runners. I opted for Karrimors again, *two* sizes too big to accommodate my swollen Hobbit feet.

Ignoring National Rail's instructions to phone ahead before using their pedestrian crossing, I negotiated the tracks and continued running in the direction of Monmouth, adding a strained left knee to my collection of injuries. In a hamlet named Three Ashes I came across an old church. The idea of throwing out my sleeping bag and being comfortably asleep by the time it hit the church's worn parquet floor was certainly appealing – only God had locked the door.

A few miles up the lane I arrived at a small patch of grass hidden from the road behind someone's back fence. Having set up camp I tried to eat a sandwich while listening to a Joe Rogan podcast but woke up at 5am with said snack still in my hand and the three-hour chat long since finished.

Day 29 | Three Ashes to Tockington | 41 Miles

The super-light Mammut sleeping bag had kept me more than warm, which was a great start to the day, especially as the tent was covered in frost. On the down side I experienced a crushing tiredness and my right ankle, for reasons unknown, had doubled in size. I ate a flapjack, packed up and then dashed into a patch of woodland to ... *punch* a bear. Then I reopened my pack and unfurled the tent as I'd left my bandana inside it.

Further along the country lane, I came across an entrance with no less than *four* signs announcing 'Meredith Farm Camping. Dr Neil Wheeler.' The good doctor had even painted his mobile number on them. Had I happened upon this land of milk and honey last night – an interesting meeting of agriculture, poultry, dairy, healing and 4G – I could have slept soundly, safe in the knowledge that should a medical emergency arise I had a doctor on call *and* the added bonus of a milkshake with my omelette in the morning.

I ran into Monmouth on a narrow, twisting and virtually empty back lane, half shaded from the sun's dazzling rays by vibrant forest. Just as I was congratulating myself on a second day in beautiful Wales a sign appeared which read 'Welcome to Wales' and the realisation dawned Hereford is actually in England and not the Land of the Leeks as I'd always believed. Below the sign was what appeared to be a smudge of lipstick. I think in some parallel universe it was supposed to represent a dragon and a designer based in Canary Wharf probably got paid £100,000 of the Welsh taxpayers' money to come up with it. Truth is my little lad could have knocked the logo out at pre-school for the price of a Spiderman comic.

In Monmouth I treated myself to a pub breakfast at the

Royal Oak and used their outside socket to charge my phone. Pam Carver, another supporter, drove by beeping and stopped to wish me luck. I would have accepted her kind offer of food had I not been full of veggie meatballs, spaghetti and salad.

A mile out of the town I stopped in a layby to unpack the now-thawed-out tent and drape it over a five-bar gate to dry. Then I embarked on a hill that put Everest to shame. Two miles up the not-so-gradual incline I was proud of my performance, not a hint of burning quad muscles or a pant from my seasoned lungs. Four miles up and the whole of Monmouth came into view beneath a pristine sky and life seemed full-on phenomenal. After two and a half hours I was ten miles up and felt not a jot of discomfort – somewhat contrary to all my previous experience of running.

Finally as I came to the conclusion Wales is one big slope up to England, I crested the valleyside and the Severn Bridge came into view. I'd run eighteen miles straight up without a single pause. I recalled John Nash's words, 'There's quite a hill coming up, boyo.'

Hill? That was a continent!

Running towards the enormous suspension bridge I spotted a familiar face. Gavin Boyter with whom I'd run with on the twenty-four-hour race and also some of his JOGLE. He'd driven all the way from London with his fiancé Aradhna to support me.

'Great to see you guys!' I was pleased to have thirty-three miles in the bag and a running partner to accompany me into my homeland.

Gavin insisted on taking the bergen, an honourable gesture considering I don't think he'd run with such weight before. Aradhna was a great fun girl. She agreed to drive their camper van and meet us in a pub in the village of Tockington, seven miles away. Gavin and I set off over the bridge at an eight-minute-mile pace. In the dark the floodlights on the bridge added an additional aura of excitement to what was essentially a mental milestone. Cars roared past and the two of us didn't spare the horses until arriving in the lounge of the Swan Inn, where Gavin and Aradhna treated me to a delicious fish supper and a much-appreciated pint.

While Gavin paid the bill I began kitting up and wondering how much further I'd have to run before finding a place to lay my head for the night. Aradhna spoke to the landlady about possible camping spots in the area and upon hearing of my efforts the women marched over and insisted I put my tent up in the beer garden. *Result!*

Day 30 | Tockington to Yatton | 26.13 Miles

During my morning update I was able to tell supporters I was on track to achieve my goal of an ultramarathon-a-day average. I also announced I had a 'special' guest running with me when I reached Bristol later in the day.

'So are you going to run with your daddy, Haz?' I asked the three-year-old I hadn't seen for a month.

Harry lunged for his red Spiderman daypack and scrambled out of the car. I pressed the video button on my phone and filmed the highlight of the trip so far – me running with my son across a park.

It was an unanticipated rendezvous. Following an early morning call to Jenny she had embarked on the six-hour-return journey from Plymouth to bring me my back support – a precautionary measure due to the steadily increasing pain I was experiencing. It was the longest we'd all been away from each other and our reunion felt a mix of special and strange. Following a meal in the Wellington pub we family-hugged and went our separate ways.

Former Royal Marine Mike 'Buster' Keating had been a constant source of support on Facebook. He messaged me to ask if there was anything I needed now that I'd stepped foot on his home turf. 'Got somewhere I can lay my sleeping bag tonight?' I inquired tentatively.

'Screw *that,* brother, you can have a double bed!' he replied, sending me his postcode in the village of Yatton.

It was three in the afternoon and sixteen miles to Buster's place. The navigator took me way off the beaten track, down country lanes not a great deal wider than my bergen, *and* in the pitch black! I couldn't see a thing without my headtorch and – *'Ooph!'* – ran smack into a drystone wall.

I made a Facebook Live update and asked for thoughts on whether I should detour south of the usual JOGLE route so people could meet me on Plymouth Hoe as I made my way through Devon. To complement the idea I began singing the Rocky theme – only for Mathew 'Fish' Peterson to point out it was actually the 'Final Countdown' by Europe.

Day 31 | Yatton to Bridgewater | 27.95 Miles

Buster and his teenage son Riley were absolute gentlemen. I don't think I've ever been appreciated so much in all my years on the planet. I'd emerged from the darkness last night into the light bathing Buster's smart detached house. My Royal Marine brother wasn't at all pushy and immediately recognised this was about *my* needs and not his.

Bath – *check!*

Dressing gown and shorts – 'Here ya go!'

Ice – *big* bag in the fridge!
Vegetable stir fry – *in* the wok!
Beer – *'Why* not!'
Spotless bedding – *et voilà!*
'Anything else you need, Chris?'
'Zzzzzzzz ...'

Following our breakfast of champions Buster looked ill at ease.

'What is it, mate?'

'Well ... I was wondering if I could run with you for a bit?' the bricklayer replied.

I assumed as Buster hadn't run for twenty-five years he meant a mile or two down the road.

'Dude, of course!'

'Yes!'

While Buster pulled on Riley's trainers, a size too small, I made a social media post asking if any of the serving marines on the page worked at the Commando Training Centre in Lympstone. And if so could they arrange for a couple of recruits to come and run with me as I approached Exeter. I figured it would be a great experience for them and equally as rewarding for me.

'I'll take the bergen,' said Buster.

'Nah, it's too heavy, mate.'

'Give!'

'Okay ...'

I helped him into the straps, figuring that with zero fitness and ill-fitting shoes Buster might last ten minutes before handing me my house back.

Approaching mid-morning we passed what looked to be an

enormous sewage plantation, a field full of round frothing ponds, each with a set of spinning arms above them. I spotted a sign for Thatcher's Cider and realised these small lakes contained fermenting apple juice. What surprised me more was when I checked the tracker Buster and I had only covered *five* miles! It honestly felt as if we'd run a half marathon – perhaps due to our engrossing conversation.

'Do you want me to take the bergen, Buster?'

'Nah.' He stared dead ahead.

We continued along the Strawberry Line, a gem of a footpath previously a railway track. It brought us out at a petrol garage. 'Mac' MacGregor was waiting there to surprise us. 'Hello Royal!' he said. 'I'm literally on my way to the airport for work but wanted to wish you good luck.'

As we entered the Orchard Inn in West Huntspill twenty miles later the bergen was still firmly on Buster's shoulders. He'd declined my offer to take it on so many occasions now that I'd long-since stopped asking. Upon hearing of our mission the Orchard's wonderful proprietor Linda Allen served up a huge plate of cheese-and-cucumber sandwiches. Talk about *perfect* timing! This magnificent effort by Buster was the most fun I'd had on the trip. Such a kind and genuine man and not a single whimper.

After a whopping thirty miles we entered the outskirts of Bridgewater and I spotted a Premier Inn. I honestly didn't mind putting the tent up – actually looked forward to it – but I wanted to go for some food with Buster to celebrate his mammoth effort before it got too late to ask his father to come and pick him up.

I walked into the Premier Inn's reception, curious to hear what the motel chain's response would be if I asked them to support our suicidal veterans by giving me a small discount.

Let's be clear here. They're a multi-million-pound company and ten percent off the room rate would cost them eleven pounds of their precious profit. In return they'd gain some great publicity *and* the respect of the public *and* help save lives.

Forty-five minutes and *several* phone calls from the receptionist to various upline managers later I was still waiting in reception shivering in my shorts. Finally the regional manager rang back to say Premier Inn supported their own charity and therefore weren't willing to offer me a reduced rate.

I hadn't asked Premier Inn to support my charity. I'd asked them to help save the lives of suicidal veterans ... and they'd refused.

Steve

I got ninety-nine problems but running ain't one.

Fireman Sam

Day 32 | Bridgewater to Red Ball | 26.24 Miles

Last night ended up being emotional – in the best possible way. My Royal Marines brother kindly paid the £110 Premier Inn charge, freeing us up to go for a pint and some grub. Steve Sellman my recruit buddy who'd sponsored me £500 turned up at the pub and immediately left for the nearby petrol station to grab me some supplies – all of which he paid for without question.

My legs were now in a bad way. Both the left knee and right ankle were still double-sized, the stress fracture in my shin unlikely to start healing until I reached Land's End. Fluid had accumulated in my calves, which now resembled tree trunks. I worried what with the pounding my body was receiving and the pain and anti-inflammatory medication I was taking that my internal organs might be struggling. My mood remained at 100% though.

Steve had thoughtfully brought some high-strength CBD oil. Back at the room he patiently massaged it into my lower limbs. Steve told me that while doing some research around my JOGLE attempt he'd come across a running forum in which one of the world's top endurance athletes had been asked, 'Is it possible to run from John O'Groats to Land's

End?'

According to Steve the guy replied, 'Pretty much impossible unless ...' and then went on to list what he felt were the – virtually superhuman – mental, physical and logistical requirements. These included an intensive five-year training regime of running, swimming, cycling and gym work, meditation and visualisation, complex route planning, a leading-edge support crew made up of sports scientists, masseurs, physiotherapists, nutritionists, a chef and drivers, along with a state-of-the-art runner's wardrobe and equipment.

It's this sensationalist and ego-fuelled nonsense that puts people off following their dreams. My 'shove your trainers on and go' approach was testament to that – although I wouldn't recommend carrying a hefty rucksack and running an ultramarathon a day. For someone who's not in the right place mentally and prepared to navigate the pain threshold it would be inviting disaster.

The passageway door in the Premier Inn banged all night long and kept me awake despite my exhausted state. In the morning I made a heartfelt video message to the supporters to express my pride and gratitude towards my Royal Marines brothers. I'd never met Buster before and yet we cracked on like family. To see him fighting through the exhaustion yesterday without a single complaint – and all to support me and my cause – was deeply special. He'd paid for all of our food and drinks too.

The same goes for Steve, who'd popped out of the ether when I'd needed it the most. Both lads had lent me their enormous support. In defiance of her spineless employers the girl on reception insisted on sending me for a free breakfast, which proved a great start to another long day.

I continued on through Somerset and thanks to Steve's efforts the swelling in my legs had reduced. Following my morning tot of rum I could handle the pain of a fractured shin, swollen ankle and busted knee but the IT bands on the outsides of my knees had become a real problem. I could only run for a quarter of a mile before having to stop and massage them for thirty seconds.

I wasn't too bothered. It was an amazing feeling to only have a few days left of the challenge. I'd soon be in Cornwall and greeting my dear little boy at Land's End – making good my promise from the start. It's impossible to put into words the feeling of sticking to your plan and seeing a dream come true.

Looking back at my progress I could now understand the pros and cons of running solo and unsupported. When setting off I genuinely believed arriving at Land's End twenty days later on my birthday was a realistic target. I'd bargained on fifty to sixty miles a day as an average. This would be easily achievable had I paired up with someone in a campervan, only by opting to do it alone you face a number of constraints.

For a start most end-to-enders don't attempt #999miles – they opt for the shorter 700-mile route. Then there's the hours spent faffing around trying to find a suitable camp spot, putting up the tent, drying equipment and organising new shoes. You have to liaise with the charity and family and supporters via endless texts and calls ... buy or order and wait for food ... cook and make drinks ... find shops to purchase ice and come up with ingenious ways to strap it to your body ... spend two hours a day charging your phone ... double check the route ... fiddle with technology ... update social media ... deal with injuries ... find a suitable place to cross roads and let traffic pass ... engage in polite chats with locals and proprietors

... message donators to say thank you ... sort out and fix equipment ... attend to personal hygiene and other admin ... not to mention navigating or taking a wrong turn. The list is endless and not only that but most unsupported runners book hotels every night and don't have to carry heavy camping gear.

I didn't know Somerset well but pressed on down the single carriageway A38 aiming for Plymouth. Being Wednesday the thought occurred to me I might make Land's End by Sunday. If so then folks could come and cheer me home. *That* would be amazing!

But what if I arrived at silly o'clock on Saturday night when everyone was tucked up in bed? I wasn't looking for fame and adulation, but it seemed a shame to have put so much effort in, raising thousands of pounds, garnering so much support and raising people's spirits, only to finish in the dark on my own. There'd be no media coverage and subsequent exposure for the Baton and the military suicide epidemic.

Hmmh ...?

I began to run through possible end scenarios that would allow me to complete the JOGLE on Saturday night and yet still meet the press and well-wishers the next day. How about camping a mile from the finish and waiting for everyone to arrive? What about actually *finishing* in the dark and then backtracking to cross the line a second time for the TV and social media cameras? That way I wouldn't add an extra day to my result.

Acht!

Que sera sera.

At the twenty-mile mark came the patter of not-so-tiny feet. I turned to see Alan Rowe, founder of the Baton, dressed in running clobber and pulling alongside me. This was a *hoofing* effort because Alan had been battling some extremely serious health issues.

'Ha-ha!' I slowed to a trot.

'Hello, mate.' Alan beamed and gave me a big hug. 'It's unbelievable what you've achieved. You've inspired *so* many people!'

'No, *they've* inspired me, Al.'

Alan and I were joined by Nigel 'Chas' Fowler, another unpaid director of the charity, who ran *backwards* whilst filming proceedings on an expensive gimbal-mounted camera. Nige was also full of praise for my efforts, but neither needed to be. You've got to do *something* with your life and going for a little jog ain't a bad option.

In a joint video update I told my now 2,500-strong band of Facebook supporters how as a barber Alan had cut the hair of veterans whose service went back to World War II. When I handed the phone over to my fellow presenter he informed our audience it was actually World War *I!*

At the twenty-five-mile mark we stopped at the Beambridge pub and Alan got the beers in plus an additional cup of tea for me. As I was getting to know more about Alan and Chas and their work with the Baton, Steve Sellman came through the door. His farm was a stone's throw away and I vaguely remembered asking him the previous evening if I could stay the night. After a great four-way catch-up, pepping me up for the final leg, Steve ran a couple more miles with me before returning for his car. I relaxed in the passenger seat, utterly contented, knowing Steve was my brother and his home was my home.

Day 33 | Red Ball to Moretonhampstead | 35 Miles

Steve has to be one of the most generous, genuine and open-minded men I've ever met. What he can tell you about the world, the *real* world and not the mainstream media puppet show, is beyond most people's comprehension. I love spending time with him.

During commando training, in the boxing, or 'milling', Steve had to fight the hardest guy in our troop. 'How you doing, mate?' I'd asked him beforehand.

'I'm *fucking* terrified ...' He'd stared into space.

Steve then entered the ring and knocked his opponent senseless!

My brother fed and watered me, washed my kit and leant moral support as I lanced an eight-day-old heel blister. Despite me covering it with a second-skin plaster the wound had grown to encompass the whole of my heel. Leaving the plaster in place I repeatedly shoved a needle through the half-golf-ball-sized dome until golden-brown puss began spewing out. It smelt rancid – a sign my foot had become infected – but other than draining the swelling there was not a lot else I could do. If I attempted to remove the plaster it would rip all the skin from my heel and the subsequent pain between here and Land's End could prove a game-changer. Then Steve wrapped me in a blanket in front of a roaring fire – and *boy* did I sleep well!

After a breakfast of organic local produce Steve drove us back to the main road, left his car in a layby and grabbed the backpack.

'Are you sure, mate?'

Although Steve was a hands-on farmer (and also a

successful businessman) who spent several weeks a year in Norway snowboarding and dogsledding, he hadn't run particularly far in years and certainly not carrying a bergen.

... I watched as he flew off down the road.

A car pulled into the layby and one of my wonderful supporters Sarah Sanders stepped out. 'I've made a donation,' she said. 'I just wanted to come and say well done!'

It was a wonderful start to another long day. As Steve and I powered down the A38 towards Exeter a motorbike roared up and a chap lifted his visor and introduced himself as Chad Harry Maskers, a former bootneck who I recognised from his relentless support on my social media pages. 'Chris I'm following you today. *Anything* you need just say the word.'

'Thanks bud,' I replied, pleased to put yet another name to a Facebook profile.

Steve's brother Wayne turned up in his truck, adding to my growing entourage, as did 'Knocker' White, a former Royal Marines colour sergeant and now a patron of the Baton. Knocker proudly wore the charity's T-shirt. Following introductions the three of us fell into a fairly fast pace. I had to ask the boys not to run in front of me as for some weird psychological reason it sapped me of adrenaline and made the going harder.

In what seemed no time we were running past the craggy tors, swaying grasses, rich green gorse and vivid purple heather of Dartmoor National Park, passing bleating sheep and the famous shaggy wild ponies. In the village of Moretonhampstead on the delightfully quiet B3212 we stopped at the Horse Pub having clocked up thirty-five miles. I felt slightly guilty as not carrying the bergen had allowed me to push pace a couple of times. Steve would never complain though. He'd kept his head down and my spirits up, and

Knocker did me proud too.

I checked my social media while the boys sorted out food. The charity total was over £8,000, *unbelievable,* with some of the contributions coming from friends I hadn't seen since school. A Royal Marine from the Commando Training Centre had messaged to say they'd received permission from on high for a couple of nods to come and join me – which was obviously too late now.

I finished my food and was about to thank the boys for their efforts and continue across the moor when Steve approached brandishing a key. 'Got you a room, mate.' He grinned.

This was a thoughtful offer I couldn't refuse. I slept in soft white comfort in one of the White Hart Hotel's quaint little rooms and saddled back up for 7.30am.

Day 34 | Moretonhampstead to Clearbrook | 26.2 Miles

I stepped onto the moor in bright sunshine and so began the craziest of days, made a little crazier by a second slug of rum I treated my aching bones to. First off I called my pa as he lived on the other side of the moor. 'Bring us a cuppa, Dad?'

'Okay ...' my old man replied, sounding on the vague side of surprised. 'What about biscuits?'

'Could be good.'

It was surreal to see him pull up in his silver Golf. As I was drinking my tea Matt Wildgoose pulled up on his bike and wished me good luck. Matt was the Sergeant's Mess manager at 42 Commando Royal Marines, my old unit on the outskirts of Plymouth. Matt was on his way to work from his home high up on the moor.

Climbing the brutal hills into the Dartmoor highlands

should have required some gritting of the teeth – only I'd developed complete immunity to whatever gradient Mother Nature threw at me. I sailed up the slopes, smiling like Julia Roberts opening a pink-fur-lined box and finding a kitten inside. The day was already so hot my smock had long since gone in the pack.

As I neared the summit of one peak I heard the weirdest of offers. 'Dartmoor *Tea!* Come and get your authentic Dartmoor *Tea!*'

I came up over the rise to find my old school chum Tim Taylor and his dad. They had set a picnic table up next to Tim's works van and were offering chai and cake!

'Hello mate.' I chuckled and set my phone to record.

I handed the filming over to Tim, who told my supporters about the *best* days we had at school – which were when we weren't there. In the last two years of education, having signed the register, we would bunk off to go snorkelling and fishing in the River Tavy or into town to buy chips and play Space Invaders.

Next on the *This is Your Life* guest list was Paul Allen, an even older friend of mine. Paul and I went to scouts together back in the seventies. Last year Paul donated one of his kidneys to a mate who was on dialysis. So now as he stood on top of a tor on Dartmoor attempting to sing my praises like a ginger Julie Andrews, I put him straight. Namely that what he'd done was far more courageous than running a few miles. When Paul asked if he could do anything for me my long-awaited order for a Cornish pasty went in lightning fast.

Running across the stunning moorland landscape, the sun on my bare shoulders and Plymouth Harbour rising out of the mist in the far distance, I heard 'Hello, Royal!' I turned to see my bootneck brother Paul Mather had pulled up and was filming my progress from his car window. Paul's second home is Dartmoor as he's the warden for the military shooting ranges in the area. It was a special moment to see him.

Little did I know but three more camera lenses lay in wait to ambush me. Hazel Mansell-Greenwood stood behind the first, snapping some truly professional shots. Hazel had a fascinating story to tell me, one which tied in with what I was saying at the Commando Memorial about the selfless men who went behind enemy lines – often on a one-way ticket – during the Second World War. Hazel's uncle was Corporal George Sheard Royal Marines, one of Blondie Hasler's Cockleshell Heroes. George drowned as a result of hypothermia while carrying out that daring canoe mission which cost the lives of eight of the ten men who took part.

The second lens pointed out of a transit van's sliding door and as the vehicle flew past I spotted ITV Westcountry News' logo emblazoned on its side. The driver pulled up a quarter of a mile ahead and a cameraman hopped out to set up for a long shot.

As I ran into frame, attempting to project the look of a grizzled but determined long-distance runner, my old mate Martin 'Smudger' Smith overtook me, his puppy on a lead, his mobile phone on record. Within seconds everything had gone Laurel and Hardy as we became one big entanglement of fur, dog leash and Android technology – all of which went out on the six o'clock news!

When I arrived at the one-sheep hamlet of Postbridge, a place I'd last visited on our survival exercise in recruit training, ITV's effervescent Jacquie Bird waited microphone in hand to interview me. All things considered it wasn't a bad bit of promotion – even though the rum let Jacquie have the veterans' plight with both barrels.

Paul Allen returned with my pasty and suggested I chuck the bergen in his car for the afternoon. I had another slug of pirate poison and continued south, backpack-free, clad only in shorts and trainers and enjoying the glorious sun.

Another runner pulled up beside me without saying anything. I glanced left and grinned. 'Hello mate!'

Pete Devlin was a good friend of mine from Plymouth and the fact he'd come to support me despite being injured spoke volumes for his character. As Pete peeled off after five miles a third lens zoomed in on me from the passenger-side window of a black Toyota – *our* Toyota! In my increasingly worse-for-wear state I briefly made out former Royal Marine Matt Elliot, the legendary photographer, as Jenny drove him and Harry off into the distance.

A little way down the road the combination of alcohol and an 850-mile bimble began to make life seem somewhat soft around the edges. For the first time since John O'Groats the enormity of what I'd put my body through saw me sink to all fours on the verge and take a moment.

A mosquito-like whine descended.

I raised my head off my arms and glanced up to see a drone hovering overhead. Ordinarily I would have laughed at the idea of Matt having eyes on me, but too smashed I threw a victory sign instead. The iconic photo, 'Pain', would later win an award – however, 'Pissed' would have been a more appropriate title.

Descending into civilisation and Dousland village I had the honour of former Royal Navy field gunner Rob Hayman's company. Rob was the first recipient of the Baton Trophy for services to the charity and had caught up with me on his bike. Haz, Jenny and Matt were waiting in the car park of the Burrator Inn and so it turned into one big JOGLE jamboree.

After a quality twenty minutes with my girl and little boy I ran on in the direction of Plymouth, knowing I'd see them both on the Hoe later.

I hadn't planned on getting waylaid at the next pub on the route. I'd known Gary Tromans and Gavin Chapple since childhood. They sat with a load more of our gang in the roadside beer garden of Yelverton's Rock Hotel. I don't remember the conversation that took place – only that everything seemed a bit rowdy for a while.

Before I knew it I was alone again and enjoying running along the cycle path next to Sir Francis Drake's Leat. Despite having run almost a marathon already I had no doubt I would make the city centre, thirteen miles away. Then Paul phoned to tell me the meeting on the Hoe had been arranged for 6pm – in twenty minutes time – and not 9pm as I'd thought. We agreed he'd pick me up from the village of Clearbrook, three miles away, so I didn't keep people waiting for hours. I'd have to ask Jenny to drop me back in the morning.

Day 35 | Clearbrook to Liskeard | 29 Miles

I awoke on the couch – *our* couch, which felt surreal. I guess I must have drifted off into oblivion after yesterday's exertions.

'Breakfast hun?' Jenny called through from the kitchen.

'Boiled egg, marmite on toast and a *big* salad, please.'

I began hunting for a pair of trainers to replace the ones John Nash bought me in Hereford. I couldn't get my swollen feet into my newest shoes and had to settle for an old pair of Karrimors. Something about them didn't feel comfortable but I had to get back on the road.

I genuinely appreciated my reception last night on the Hoe and the efforts of the folks who'd turned out – my dad, brother Ben, sister Becky, Matty Elliot, Paul Allen, Plymouth Mary, former marine Andy Stuart and old friends Bungy and Debs – and the detour south to Plymouth had helped me towards my target of #999miles.

Back at Clearbrook I joined the National Cycle Route, which runs along the old steam train tracks on the wooded banks of the River Plym. I left the trail at Bickleigh as there was a tribute I wanted to make to Marine Adam 'Gilly' Gilbert, shot dead in the early days of our Northern Ireland tour.

Killer Hill is the infamous stretch of lane leading up to 42 Commando's Bickleigh Barracks, the unit Gilly and I had served with. The gradient of this torturous quarter mile needs no further elucidation. Back in the day us young marines feared running up this beast more than death itself. Yet now, having put on my green beret as a sign of respect for Gilly and the men of Lima Company, I didn't even break a sweat, sailing up the forty-five-degree slope with ease whilst making a Facebook Live broadcast. If you'd told the ballbagged teenage me I'd be cruising up Killer Hill at half a century old, carrying a bergen and talking on the phone, I'm not entirely sure I would have believed you.

As I continued along Bickleigh Lane towards the city a chap past me on his bike, did a double take and stopped. 'You're *that* guy!' He grinned.

'Hah!' I smiled for his selfie.

I'd not long turned off the lane when a car heading in the direction of the barracks pulled up and the driver shouted, 'Royal!'

'Hello, brother.' I hopped in the passenger seat.

'Ash' introduced himself. 'I thought it was you. Anything you need from the camp – a coffee or something?'

'That would be amazing, Ash, thanks.' I felt like royalty.

'Cool and I'll grab you a pasty.'

Ash's gesture meant the world and to have serving members of the Corps supporting my efforts felt extremely rewarding. Ash was a member of the British bobsleigh team and he invited me to join them in the Alps for a spot of training.

On the edge of the city I stopped by my old house and took a photo of the street sign. Carroll Road is where the events in my memoir 'Forty Nights' took place, the story of how the lessons I learned from extreme adversity allowed me to smash all my goals and live in paradise. There are no positive experiences and no negative experiences, only experiences – and you can't master your life without them.

The Tamar Bridge between Devon and Cornwall loomed in the distance – as did Carl Brough, a bootneck brother waiting to wish me luck. After a brief chat I ran onwards but was stopped by the beep of a car horn. Steve Wilkes, a former sailor, and his wife Lynn flagged me down and tucked a tenner in my hand, going on to explain how a veteran's suicide had affected them personally.

Then *there* was the majestic suspension bridge, the gateway to the Land of Milk and Honey, aka Cornwall, and my final destination Land's End! I took a selfie to thank my amazing supporters and ran across the impressive span. At Landrake I left the A38 in the darkness and headed off down the back lanes, a ten-mile-long shortcut I used to rally through in the eighties in my souped-up Ford Escort. I couldn't remember the exact route and had to rely on the satnav and signposts, which added an element of uncertainty and unease in the pitch black.

Approaching midnight, headlights picked me out, which

had to be old bill. A blonde-haired officer named Kim stopped to ask if I was okay. Following a photo together I soon found myself back on the A38 at Liskeard. The enormous dual-carriageway appeared barren and the out-on-a-limb feeling I'd experienced the night I slept in the yurt returned. It's funny how you can feel lonely on a major British highway but not in an empty country lane while unable to see your hand in front of your face.

I had half a litre of water and no food and felt unsure about continuing for fear there might not be services for miles. If I sought out a camping spot for the night I could at least backtrack a mile into Liskeard town centre in the morning and grab some supplies. I left the deserted tarmac and climbed up the embankment, pitching my tent in a copse behind a row of houses. It was Saturday tomorrow and roughly eighty miles to Land's End. Had I been experiencing less pain and exhaustion I might have realised I could be there at some point on Sunday. It would mean ignoring the agony in my knees and banging out *two* forty milers. But instead I drifted off to sleep in my Mammut bag and enjoyed the driest night so far.

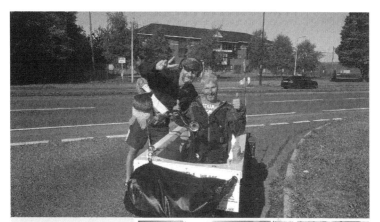

In the bath with legendary charity fundraiser Stuart Kettell, also en route to Land's End.

Happy 49th birthday to me – thank you Cath Green and family for the amazing hospitality.

Timeout – Hereford.

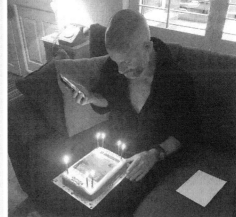

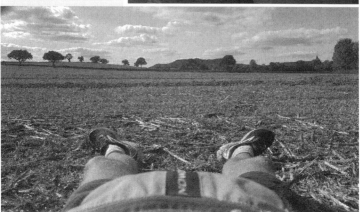

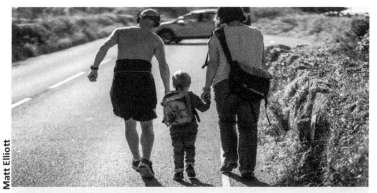

Family – with Jenny and Harry.

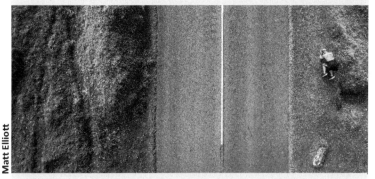

P****d!

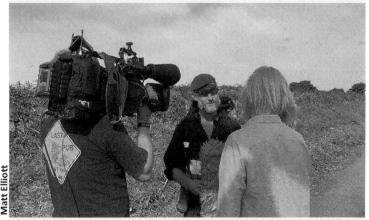

With the BBC on the final stretch into Land's End.

My Boy

You get one life – SMASH it!

Chris Thrall

Day 36 | Liskeard to Redruth | 43 Miles

In the morning I stood on the edge of the A38 watching the enormous carriageway disappear into the distance. *Do I take the safe bet and backtrack to Liskeard for food and water?*

I couldn't bring myself to turn around. There had to be somewhere to refuel within twenty miles and I could last without food and only half a litre of the wet stuff until then. It wasn't as if I was heading into the Empty Quarter on an emaciated camel under the merciless Arabian sun. I could have checked the Internet but was too exhausted to think let alone operate fiddly and frustrating technology. It was easier to point south and put one foot in front of the other, a system that had worked well for me across three countries – or four if you're a member of the Cornish Liberation Army.

It was A roads all the way to Land's End – only these bad boys were dual-carriageways with super-fast long straights. I may as well have been on a motorway, the cars hurtling past at ridiculous speeds as I shuffled along the hard shoulder. Although I wasn't breaking any law it did feel a bit weird and I knew it was only a matter of time before some jobsworth driver reported me to the police for daring to exit the Matrix and steer my own path through life.

One of the walkers I'd met at John O'Groats told me the

cops had escorted him off the highway in Cornwall. If they tried to spring that unlawful nonsense on me it would end up like a scene from *First Blood* – and I don't mean the bit where Johnny Rambo spears a wild boar with a sharpened boy scout.

My knee pain had reached an all-time high, likewise the total for the Baton charity, which now stood at £10,000. If I could make Land's End by tomorrow afternoon and get some media exposure this would surely add to the pot. Albeit only a tick-box amount over the fabled marathon distance, I'd averaged thirty-five ultras to date, 920 miles, despite my growing catalogue of injuries. If I was to achieve my goal of an ultramarathon a day average I'd have to limit tonight's sleep to three hours and run the remaining eighty odd miles in little more than a day.

You've got this ...

I adjusted the straps on my bergen for the five-thousandth time and began heading south.

A sign for Dobwalls appeared and so I veered off the main road to search for food and charge the phone. I entered a Spar shop and found to my surprise the manager was Luke, a chap I used to work with. I plugged the charger in and rested the phone on a stack of the *Cornish Times,* then bought sandwiches and snacks and chatted to my old pal. The Samsung S7 Edge had proved to be a great asset, its battery lasting twenty-four hours and the video and audio superb. The only design flaw was the camera lens, which for some unknown reason made me appear devastatingly handsome and risked triggering an avalanche of marriage proposals from sex-crazed Scandinavian nurses – but that's technology for you.

It felt as if the cushioning had gone in my old trainers. I played around with various combinations of insoles, including the ones Matt had bought me in Ludlow. Nothing worked though and I became increasingly concerned I might pick up another injury or exacerbate my existing ones. Jenny went to Sports Direct in Plymouth City Centre and when she mentioned what I was doing the manager sold the shoes to her at cost – *screw* Premier Inn!

And so ensued another unanticipated meeting with my girlfriend and son, this time in a layby near Trago Mills – Cornwall's number-one discount centre for chairs, tables and beds ... *and* industrial-strength oven cleaner. I'd given Jenny instructions to buy me exactly the same pair of Karrimors as the worn-out ones I'd left at home, but when I opened the box my heart dropped – they were a different style *and* a strange fit.

My former marine buddy Tom and his partner Lou lived in Cornwall. I'd planned to stay with them tonight if possible, but the couple were away tackling a Paris to Dakar banger rally. Tom's parents turned up to wish me well though, only I was too preoccupied sorting my footwear out to give them my complete attention. I now had double-insoled shoes which were neither comfortable or uncomfortable. Moving off down the road I put the disappointment out of my mind and instead focused on my footfall to avoid worsening my back, blisters and stress fracture.

So far this trip all the people who said they were coming to run with me hadn't and those who did had done so unannounced and without drama. Today's self-preservation efforts involved stepping up onto banks, blending into hedges and sprinting across the road to avoid oncoming traffic on the perilous bends. Therefore, in view of the increasing amount of location requests, I made a Facebook video post asking fellow runners not to join me until I reached Penzance as I lacked the mental energy to worry about anyone's welfare other than my own.

The A38 turned into the A30, hopefully the last stretch of road I would use on this trip. I was unfamiliar with the names I saw on signposts because the relatively new carriageway bypassed all the towns I remembered from childhood holidays. Sticking with the hard shoulder I ran along the super highway, hemmed in by newly forested embankments or surrounded by rolling farmland dotted with towering white wind turbines. Every time a junction appeared I took time to cross the off and on ramps safely as I didn't want to add unnecessary distance to my journey by skirting the overhead roundabouts.

A large service station popped up on the opposite side of the carriageway. I ran across four lanes of busy traffic and hopped the central reservation to reach it. Time was now my enemy and so for only the second time in twenty years I entered a McDonald's and ordered coke and a fish burger.

Sitting there with my phone on charge, kids squabbling over Happy Meals, parents mopping up spilt drinks, I chuckled. Instead of being an ultra-endurance athlete on a life-saving mission, inspiring others and raising over ten thousand pounds in the process, to my fellow eaters I was a heavily tanned and scruffy bearded homeless bloke clad in a torn smock, faded bandana and overly large running shoes.

As I continued south blue-flashing lights and a siren erupted and a police car skidding to a halt on the hard shoulder. 'Are you alright, mate?' asked one of two male coppers who sprang from the fluorescent-striped criminal catcher. 'What are you doing?'

'Running to Land's End.'

'From where?' He raised an eyebrow.

'John O'Groats.'

'Really?

'It's just that we've had *five* phone calls from the public.' His partner chuckled.

'Yeah, because a guy in *shorts* and *trainers,* carrying a *dayglo* backpack and heading *south* on the A30 couldn't *possibly* be on his way to Land's End for charity!' I grinned.

'Hah!'

The officers wished me luck and sped off to investigate reports of a 'rosy-cheeked bloke driving a big red thing full of turnips' and some 'orange-and-white-striped pointy objects in the middle of the road'.

Next up for company was former Royal Marine Pincher Martyn. Pinch came bounding down the hard shoulder towards me, his wife driving on ahead in their car. 'Hoofing effort Chris!' He tucked fifty quid in my hand. 'Most special forces operators would struggle to do what you've done.'

Pinch's words were rewarding. Having already made a generous donation to the charity, he stressed the fifty quid was for me to grab a hotel room. Pinch ran with me for an hour until darkness fell. Then I continued into the night, pleased when the A30 changed to a single carriageway and the flow of cars thinned. There was nowhere to run except on the road and so I put my headtorch on – although this did nothing to deter pretty much every car driver dazzling me with their full beam.

As I came off a roundabout a four-by-four sat parked on the verge. 'Chris,' shouted its driver, 'Alec Savery.'

Unsure of my exact location Alec had waited patiently for my arrival and come armed with a flask of coffee and a sandwich. Over the next twenty minutes Alec explained how he knew my efforts had inspired individuals suffering from the often-incapacitating effects of trauma.

By 11pm I'd covered around thirty-five miles and had no intention of stopping. Every metre I clocked up would make tomorrow's finale easier – even though it *was* almost tomorrow. In the light of my headtorch I made a Facebook update video urging others to follow their dreams by adopting a simple philosophy and straightforward action planning. I gave the example of the defeatist attitude almost always adopted by the England football team – 'If we get a bit of luck ... If the ball goes our way' – highlighting how this 'lost before we've begun' approach isn't helpful for anyone.

About eight miles from Redruth blue lights erupted once again on the dual carriageway.

Oh, for fucks sake!

What with the police in these parts still working overtime solving the 1978 'Mystery of the Missing Pasty' I reckon my little jaunt was creating a two-year backlog for them.

My cursing couldn't have been more unwarranted for I met the epitome of great British policing in the form of Marie Moore, who pulled up in a van with her partner Craig. 'You're the *guy!*' Marie yelled and beamed from the driver's seat. *'Everyone* at the station is talking about you!'

The delightful pair wouldn't stop singing my praises and were clearly in awe of what I'd accomplished. Craig, who'd reached Week 24 of commando training before being medically discharged, was particularly impressed with my efforts.

'Where are you staying tonight?' asked Marie.

'In the tent.'

'No! Stay at ours. My hubby Stuart was a Royal Marine.'

It was a touching offer and being treated as a VIP by the police was a bit of a spinner.

I continued onwards with Marie's number on my phone just in case, but at three in the morning Stuart rolled up in his jeep to check I was okay. With forty-three miles in the bank my knees decided to call it a night and I hopped in beside him.

Day 37 | Redruth to Land's End | 31 Miles

Stuart woke me with a cup of tea at 6.30am.

I'd had three hours sleep. A plate of fish-finger sandwiches and a bottle of beer lay virtually untouched next to the bed. I'd been too tired to eat or drink last night and had declined Stuart's thoughtful offer to wash my clothes – which now stank of alcohol, pain meds and stale sweat – because I didn't have the energy to think. All I wanted to do was point in the direction of Land's End and run – everything else created a distraction and zapped my dwindling reserves.

Marie was asleep from her nightshift and so Stuart and I tiptoed out of the house and headed for a Co-op to grab a coffee. Stuart had some Ziploc bags and our plan was to fill them with ice and gaffer tape them around my knees. The Co-op had no ice though and so Stuart dropped me at the A30 and went on the hunt. I necked a tot of rum and began trotting along the hard shoulder, my backpack a kilo lighter as I no longer needed the camping gear and had therefore left it at the guys' house. Despite the pain, exhaustion and lack of sleep I felt Grade A brilliant. Today was the day I'd promised everyone I would make happen, the day I would see my son and I was going to enjoy it.

I'd covered no more than a mile when blue lights erupted and a diamond-white chase car skidded to a halt in front of me. Out jumped a puffed-up chest who had 'taking yourself too seriously' down to a fine art. 'Hold it *right* there! he ordered.

'Hold *what,* officer?'

'We've had reports of a crazy guy lying in the middle of the carriageway drinking beer.'

I thought back to the carton of coffee I'd downed at the roadside. 'I'm running to Land's End, officer.'

Wait for it ...

'Where from?'

'John O'Groats.'

'Oh ...' He eyed me warily. 'You've not been drinking, have you?'

'No,' I lied.

'And what's *this?'*

My heart dropped as he pointed at the 330ml coke bottle in the neoprene holder on my rucksack's waist strap – the one two thirds full of ... *alcohol.*

'That's –'

'Coca-Cola,' he interrupted – which was technically perverting the course of justice and I was quite within my rights to make a citizen's arrest.

'I stayed with your colleague Marie last night.' I played my get-out-of-jail-free card.

'Marie? From Redruth?'

'Yep.'

'Well, there's *no* law against running down a dual carriageway.' He shrugged. 'So good luck.'

As the officer made his way back to the vehicle he suddenly stopped and turned. 'Have you *really* run from John O'Groats?'

Stuart called to say he had the ice and would meet me at a certain junction. Something must have got lost in translation, for rather than continuing straight down the carriageway, where unbeknown to me Stu waited on an overpass, I veered off down a slip road in search of him. Finding myself in No Man's Land and to save retracing my steps, I climbed a near-vertical fifty-foot-high bank to get back to where I was in the first place.

Stuart had thoughtfully bought me a load of snacks but had been unable to find any real ice. 'I got these.' He waggled four aerosol cans of Freeze Ice.

My mood took a hit. I needed proper ice to shrink the agony in my knees. I couldn't see the spray being anywhere near as effective.

No negatives on this trip ...

I applied a liberal amount of Freeze Ice to both knees and Stuart promised to keep looking for the real McCoy. Then I set off again, accompanied by the novel feeling I would finish today and deposit a dream in the bank.

Thanks to the power of social media car horns blared every few minutes as people wished me well. When I next stopped to wait for Stuart I posted a photo of me wearing my green beret, along with a map of the JOGLE route and the caption '36 ultramarathons in 36 days. It's a state of mind', which received hundreds of thousands of views, shares and likes.

A former marine Craig Thomson and his wife Jennifer waited on the verge with a pie and a Lucozade. I couldn't believe how much enthusiasm they oozed for my efforts. It was humbling and energising and representative of the Royal Marines' family ethos. As I continued towards Land's End life became one big jamboree ... *with* hotdogs. I'm not kidding – one dear old Royal jogged up alongside and handed me a couple.

By the time I reached Penzance I felt like a VIP – although conscious of the clock because the BBC were waiting somewhere along the route to film an interview. One of my supporters, Fraser Houchen, had kindly arranged this. Knocker White returned with Alec Savery by his side. Their partners drove ahead to Land's End, as did Jenny, Harry and Matty Elliot with his camera equipment.

Ever loyal and attentive, Stuart rocked up with the avocado roll I'd requested – only I couldn't sum up an appetite. This was the only day of my journey in which the actual *running* proved hard. I was beyond spent, sleep deprived, glycogen levels depleted, the muscles in my swollen legs cramping and lacking power. Each plod felt like lead, the pain wracking my every molecule far worse than 'hitting the wall' during a marathon. My IT band damage was now so unbearable we had to stop every 200 metres and spray them with Freeze Ice.

I wasn't complaining though. I had a job to do – to meet my beautiful son Haz. I'd given my word we would run to the Land's End sign post together and there was no way José I'd ever let him down. In truth the searing agony and exhaustion couldn't touch me. On day one at John O'Groats I'd constructed a mental fortress using granite blocks of positivity cemented in place by single-minded determination, unwavering self-belief and a shovelful of man the fuck up.

My marine buddies Yosser Hughes and serving Colour Sergeant Dutchy Holland popped up every so often to cheer me on from behind an enormous Corps flag. Jay Lewis, another commando and star of my favourite angling program *Fishing Impossible,* arrived at my side to lend brotherly support. 'How's Blowfish?' I hoarsed – which is not something you get to ask every day.

If things weren't surreal enough they were about to get surrealer. As Knocker and Alec and I split from a sprawl of well-wishers and headed down the Long Rock Bypass, the

BBC film crew waited in ambush – if you can call 'completely unprepared' an ambush. Andrea the reporter wielded an enormous and expensive-looking microphone and her sidekick Jeremy a bulky state-of-the-art camera, but both appeared to be more concerned with professional bickering.

'Right, Jezzy baby, I want you running backwards, camera rolling, panning out from Chris to capture me *dashing* alongside him, *breathless,* hair a *mess,* utterly committed to *nailing* the interview at all costs,' ordered Andrea. 'Think Linda Kozlowski braving *monster* crocs in the Australian outback.'

'Can't I just point the camera at Chris and you interview him?' Jeremy looked to the sky and tutted.

'Jez, *don't* second guess me!' Andrea's face turned purple. 'I want *running!* I want *dashing!* I want *fucking* breathlessness! Have you *got* it?'

'... *But* what if I trip over and hurt myself?' Jeremy's bottom lip tremored.

'Then you're *tripping over* for the sake of *art!'*

Okay ... maybe that's not *exactly* the way the conversation went, but watching these two trying to get their act together *was* bloody hilarious. I did the interview so out of my mind with pain I could hardly get the words out. When asked how the JOGLE compared with my other adventures around the globe I s-s-s-stammered something about flying planes and jumping out of them. When I later saw the feature, though, the BBC editor had done me and the Baton charity proud.

I made a second-to-last video update in which I reminded my amazing supporters that somewhere in the UK tonight a veteran would take his or her own life and the family would have to attempt to pick up the pieces. I told the story of how a simple career development grant from the Royal British

Legion had helped me get back on my feet and go and work with those street kids in Mozambique. I urged everyone who hadn't yet donated to chuck a fiver into the pot, which now stood at almost fifteen thousand pounds.

If my endurance hadn't been put to the test over the last thirty-six days it was about to be now. Just as I'd tucked Wolfie into the chest strap of my bergen ready to hand the canine back to Haz, my veteran Royal Marines chaperones Knocker and Alec decided to escort me along the scenic seafront route to avoid the A30's lethal turns. On any other day in my life I would have relished the chance to jog along the stunning coastline. Problem was I'd mentally and physically provisioned for twenty-seven miles today. The coastal path added an extra *four* to this distance and my battered legs simply didn't have that in them.

And not only that but the off-road track we jogged along consisted of gravel, cobbles and rocks and this meant I had to both think *and* pick my feet up – which put me in the pain cave big time. I was now on fumes and so shattered that I ran past the BBC camera crew without even noticing them.

I could no longer speak - I needed the energy for my dying legs. My instructions to the boys now consisted of sign language and grunts. We sprayed my knees with Freeze Ice so many times I feared the last can would empty. *Everything* had become super annoying – the road surface, the cars whizzing by, tourists meandering across our path, the seagulls squawking overhead. As far as this callsign was concerned 'everything' could *fuck off!*

Knocker kept offering to carry the backpack but I wasn't going to take the easy option now. I asked the boys not to run in front of me as having to tag along at the back was destroying my resolve. I also told them not to try and help me over the road because attempting to control the traffic and coordinate the three of us crossing was a huge waste of time. It was better I picked my moment and dashed between the cars when the need arose.

Regardless of the extra miles the boys were brilliant and unquestionably supporting their brother. The brightly coloured fishing boats bobbing on the shimmering ocean, quaint white cottages, crashing waves and the smell of brine combined to create a memorable experience that looking back I wouldn't have swapped for anything and certainly not the more functional A30 route. I was almost at the journey's end and an achievement I could treasure for the rest of my life.

'Look, there's Michael's Mount!' Knocker attempted to divert my attention from the torture.

'Hrrrh ...'

It didn't work.

A pub appeared and unable to speak I made a beeline for its aging oak door. The boys ran on a while before realising I'd departed the ranks. Knocker bought me a much-needed pint of lime and soda. The bar staff were all over my challenge, firing questions at the boys as I sat in a trance staring at the table. So whacked out of my mind I forgot to charge the phone, which now only had five-percent battery remaining.

When the boys and I got back on the road the extra distance of our little detour hit me hard. Every time we passed a sign for the A30 I kicked myself for not insisting we ran along its smooth tarmac.

My favourite police officer Marie appeared out of nowhere clad in running gear – a kind gesture I would never forget – and as the four of us hit the back lanes my bootneck mate Nige 'Bobby' Charlton shouted good luck, whizzing past on his bike en route to Land's End to clap me in. Then another good buddy, Andy Acton from my recruit troop, popped up at the side of the road having driven all the way from the Midlands. I broke from running and dashed across the road to say hello.

'Bergen ...' I rasped at Knocker. 'Beret ... top flap.'

Out came the 'green death' and I screwed it onto my head with pride.

The first sign sprung up saying Land's End. I powered onwards, hugging the hedge on the endless blind bends, waving a hand to give the drivers as much warning of me and my entourage as possible.

And then the A30 had gone ....

I found myself on a lane in open countryside, a sprinkling of white cottages and the crashing Atlantic Ocean to my front. As the team sprayed my knees for the fiftieth time I must have been a mile from the finish.

Half a mile ...

Quarter ...

Five hundred metres –

I stopped and laughed.

On a fence post the boys had stuck a copy of the Commando Training Centre's legendary '500 Metres to Go – It's Only Pain!' sign!

Before I knew it Knocker with a deep look of gratitude had handed me the official 'baton' and the three of them sprinted off to join the welcome committee.

I felt no pain or emotion bar a deep sense of pride.

I'd promised everyone I'd run an ultramarathon a day the length of the country and that's what I'd done. I'd ignored the naysayers, believed in myself and put the needs of struggling veterans first. I'd shown the public what a Royal Marines Commando is capable of but more importantly what those of us who've experienced mental health challenges can achieve.

I'd demonstrated there is *always* a way, *always* a light – along with the importance of *embracing* change, *taking* action and *smiling* at the morning sun *every* day without fail. But most of all I'd shown my beautiful and incredible son that his daddy always puts his money where his mouth is, while steering his own path and leading from the front.

Unbeknown to me the reception committee spread all the way along the final drag. Veterans held up standards including the Royal Marines' corps crest and colours. The BBC camera crew were rolling and Matty Elliot had his drone aloft. My Jenny and dad and brother stood waiting to clap and cheer, as did Alan Rowe and fellow members of the Baton family and Ed Bolton, a chap who'd recovered from blindness to complete the JOGLE himself. There would be several folks I'd never met, along with a troop of my bootneck brothers, including Chad Harry Maskers, Jay Lewis, Andy Acton, Steve Sellman, Dutchy Holland, Yosser Hughes, Bobby Charlton and Buster Keating, many of them wearing their coveted green lids.

The sun sprayed pink and orange across an indigo sky and as I came up over a rise there was Harry waiting patiently to run the last fifty metres with me.

'Daddy!'

'Hello, *my boy!*'

The End

Epilogue

As with all the best-laid plans ... they don't work! It's tradition on the JOGLE to run and symbolically touch the famous signpost – but by the time I'd done this over half of my reception party had disappeared. I think they thought I had buggered off to the Land's End Hotel room Alan Rowe had kindly paid for!

I stood in the bar with my family and friends, yet for the first time on the trip I was shattered and only managed a pint before slipping away with Jenny and Haz to our luxurious honeymoon suite. I couldn't resist a hot bath but paid the price the next morning when I could hardly walk to the enormous breakfast Steve Sellman had generously arranged. My legs had seized and were in the most agony they'd ever been in my life.

My camera battery gave up in the middle of the Facebook Live I was broadcasting on the final stretch into Land's End and so I wandered outside to have my photo taken beneath the famous signpost – with '999 MILES 8TH OCTOBER VETERANS' written on it – and update my loyal supporters. I left them with a quote a traumatised marine had just sent me:

Where I once saw darkness, I now see light.

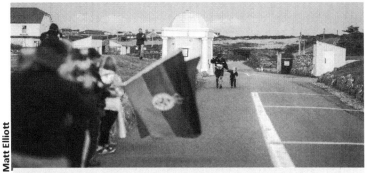

My vision for 36 days – running with my boy to Land's End.

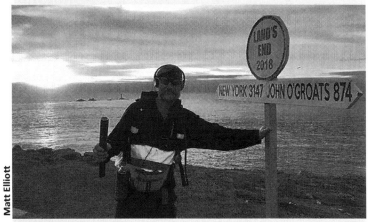

End-Ex.

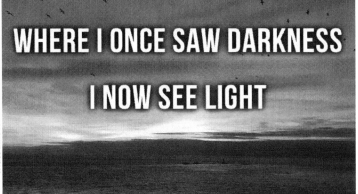

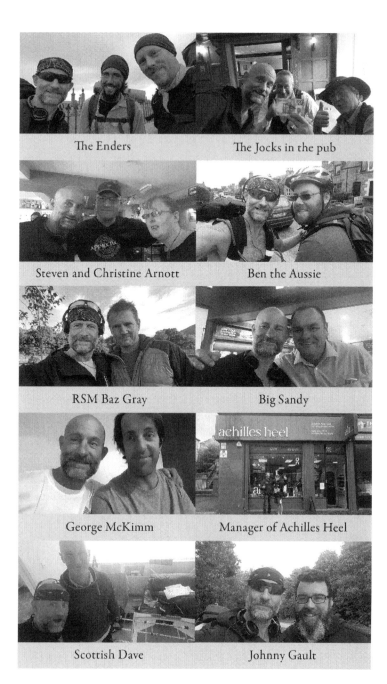

The Enders

The Jocks in the pub

Steven and Christine Arnott

Ben the Aussie

RSM Baz Gray

Big Sandy

George McKimm

Manager of Achilles Heel

Scottish Dave

Johnny Gault

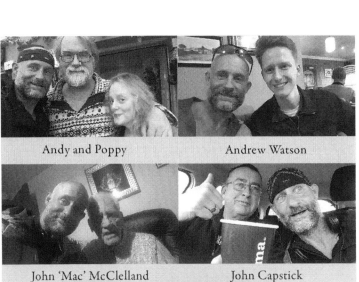

Andy and Poppy

Andrew Watson

John 'Mac' McClelland

John Capstick

Alistair and Sarah

J Wilcock, Jacki and Dolly

Tim, James and Cath Green

Neil and Drew Davies

Mathew 'Fish' Peterson

Davey and Russell 'VUAS'

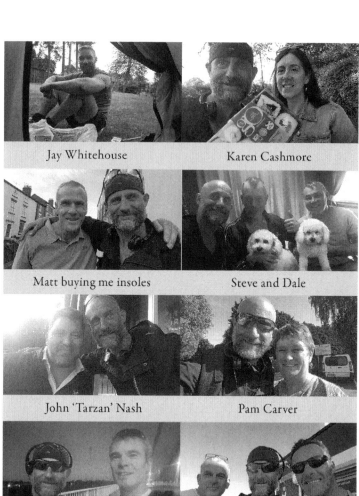

Jay Whitehouse

Karen Cashmore

Matt buying me insoles

Steve and Dale

John 'Tarzan' Nash

Pam Carver

Gavin Boyter, ultrarunner

'Mac' MacGregor and Buster

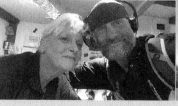

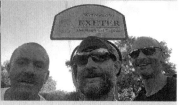

Linda Allen

Knocker and Steve Sellman

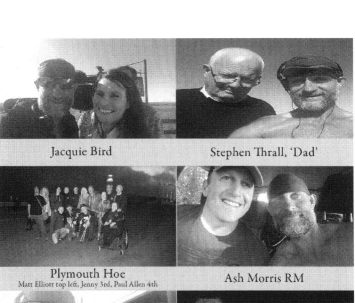

Jacquie Bird

Stephen Thrall, 'Dad'

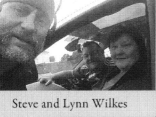

Plymouth Hoe
Matt Elliott top left, Jenny 3rd, Paul Allen 4th

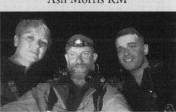

Ash Morris RM

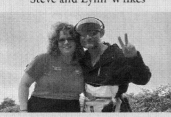

Steve and Lynn Wilkes

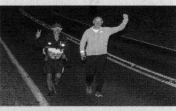

Marie Moore and Craig

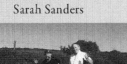

Sarah Sanders

Alan Rowe, the Baton

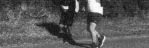

Pete Devlin

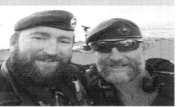

Chad Harry Maskers

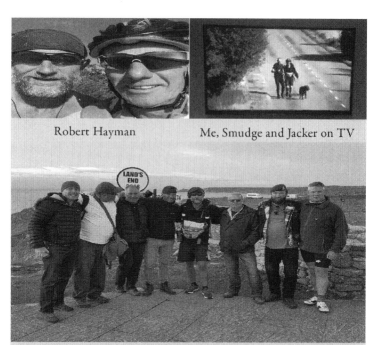

Robert Hayman   Me, Smudge and Jacker on TV

The Royal Marines Commandos
Andy Acton, Matty Elliott, Dutchy, Buster, Me, Royal, Chad, Bobby Charlton

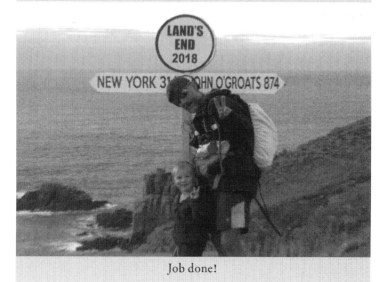

Job done!

Join My One Life TEAM

Friends, if you appreciate my writing and charity work could you please support me by joining my 'One Life TEAM' on Patreon? From as little as £1.99 a month you can begin accessing perks ranging from complimentory VIP tickets to my annual talk, e-copies of my books, insider updates, life skills tips and coaching, private monthly Q&As and TEAM and top sponsor chats, personally signed memoirs and a yearly dinner.

patreon.com/christhrall

youtube.com/christhrall

Or you can make a one-off contribution via these platforms.

paypal.me/TeamThrall

gofundme.com/christhrall

ko-fi.com/christhrall

Thank you.

Social Media

christhrall.com

patreon.com/christhrall

youtube.com/christhrall

brandnewtube.com/@christhrall

bitchute.com/christhrall

linkedin.com/in/christhrall

twitter.com/christhrall

parler.com/christhrall

facebook.com/christhrall

facebook.com/groups/christhrall

instagram.com/chris.thrall

pinterest.com/christhrall

Newsletter

Subscribe to my no-spam newsletter and receive two complimentary eBooks plus updates and life-coaching tips.

christhrall.com/mailing-list

Route

Kit List

Smart phone
Air ticket
Photo ID for flying
Debit Card
Credit Card – kept separate for emergency
Bum bag
Rucksack
Fluorescent waterproof rucksack cover
Reflectors
Backpack lights
Headtorch
Clip-on Silva compass
Phone and USB cable
Double USB fast charging plug
Ultralight tent
Ultralight sleeping bag
Ultralight mattress and repair patches
Roll-up Pillow
Woolly hat
Bandana
MP3 player
Head phones
Breathable waterproof jacket
Breathable waterproof trousers
Ultralight fleece
Tracksters
Spare socks
Running shoes x 4

Shorts
Neoprene drinks bottle holder
Water bladder
Water sterilisation tablets
Tissue
Small square of camping towel
Anti-inflammatories
Painkillers
Blister plasters
Toothbrush and paste
Wet-wipes
Sunglasses
Cushioned insoles

ITEMS I DITCHED OR SENT HOME

Loose pages from an AA road map
Lightweight grab bag for tech and in-tent kit
Map case
Medical pack
Suncream
Mini tripod
Power bank
Runners gloves
T-shirts
Thermal top
Wash kit
Compression sleeves
Cooker, gas and wind shield
Cooking pot
Drinks kit
Lighter

Swiss Army knife
Spork (knife+fork+spoon)
Small pot scrubber
Small pot of washing up liquid
Mini chopping board
Mosquito repellent
Book

The Baton Charity

Total £17,621.92

The Baton is a symbol of national conscience, crafted with care and respect from the handle of a stretcher – symbolising pride, hope, courage and suffering.

Primarily set up for awareness it carries a message of gratitude from those who wish to support the brave men and women of our armed forces who have and do risk their lives so that we may live with freedom of choice, peace and safety.

Any funds donated are used for immediate and often emergency support and to assist individuals striving to improve their personal situation, the history of this can be seen on our Welfare Support page – no wages are paid and minimal expenses taken just ordinary people doing what they can simply because they care.

The Baton Family – there for serving, former serving, their families and often those who feel forgotten.

thebaton.co.uk

Sponsors

I am deeply grateful to Marc Spender and also Mark Beresford from Bootneck Money for their unreserved generosity. Bootneck Money offers financial and investment advice to serving and former Royal Marines.

bootneckmoney.com

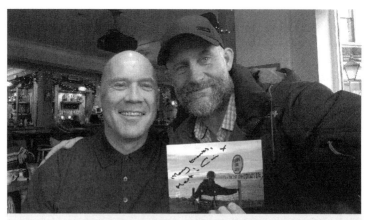

Mark Beresford from Bootneck Money

Acknowledgements

I would like to express my gratitude to everyone mentioned in this book for their kindness, generosity and support. Massive thank you to my Jenny for her total belief in me and to the wonderful Sian Forsythe at Serf Books for proofreading the manuscript. A special shout-out to Matt Elliott at MRE Photography for his spectacular images and video coverage of the event.

Books by Chris Thrall

NON-FICTION

Eating Smoke: One Man's Descent into Crystal Meth Psychosis in Hong Kong's Triad Heartland

Forty Nights: My Escape from Crystal Meth Hell

State of Mind: How I Ran 36 Ultramarathons Back to Back with No Training

How to Write a Memoir (**FREE** eBook – link on newsletter)

FICTION

The Hans Larsson thrillers

The Drift (**FREE** eBook – link on newsletter)

The Trade

Services by Chris Thrall

Inspirational Speaking

Life Coaching

Writing Guidance

Bought the T-Shirt Podcast

Please visit christhrall.com for further information

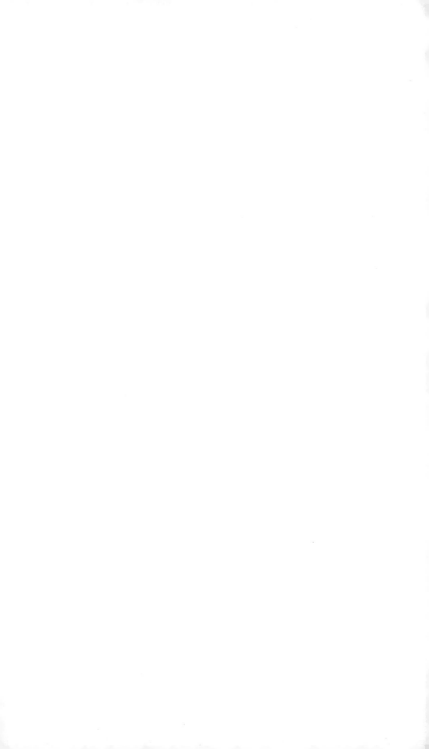

Printed in Great Britain
by Amazon